The Bible Book of Medical Wisdom

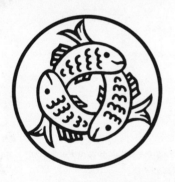

RUSSEL J. THOMSEN, M.D.

Fleming H. Revell Company
Old Tappan, New Jersey

Library of Congress Cataloging in Publication Data

Thomsen, Russel J
    The Bible book of medical wisdom.

    Includes bibliographical references
        1. Bible—Medicine, hygiene, etc.   I.   Title.
[DNLM: 1.   Medicine in literature.   2.   Religion   and   Medicine.
WZ330 T48lb]
R135.5T47   220.8'61   74–11162
ISBN 0–8007–0682–X

CONTENTS

3

Foreword

In reading medical references in the Bible, one has often wished for amplification from a twentieth-century physician. In this book Russel J. Thomsen, M.D., supplies this need with medical accuracy and interest.

He does not scoff at a Goliath over nine feet tall but even specifies the hormone causing such gigantism. Another example is the biblical description of King Jehoram's fatal illness. Outstanding theologians have read this passage but never sensed its medical accuracy—but after looking at it through Dr. Thomsen's eyes, one may well pause in reverence at its inconspicuous niceties of medical detail.

He reminds me of a guide who gave the needed appreciation of a masterpiece in a London art gallery. With his magnifying glass, I could see detailed coloring of the feathers of unnoticed fowl in a farm scene. In a similar fashion Dr. Thomsen gives one an enlarged appreciation of the beauty of scriptural exactness.

This book has another function: It points out how biblical commands saved countless thousands of lives of obedient Israelites. Through all the centuries since that time, these admonitions were often ridiculed. It was not until the birth of modern medicine that fumbling mankind even sensed the scientific reasons for these directives.

Thus, Dr. Thomsen gives sound medical substantiation for the divine inspiration of the Word.

S. I. MC MILLEN, M. D.

INTRODUCTION

The Bible comes to the present world as a book which with even the benefit of modern vernacular seems apparently disjointed. The meaning of its ancient stories escapes all but the most motivated persons—those who will spend the time to become involved in the Bible for what it claims of itself.

The Bible is not just another book with various chapters marking off action or time sequences. It is not a work of a person wherein his views are arranged in logical order. The Bible is in fact a book of books. Its authors were many, some known to us, others unknown. Its historical survey covered some hundreds of years, and its perspective covers all time. Many suspect that the Bible is a book about God. But that is wrong. Other persons look at this ancient collection of writings as literature with the usual array of poetry, short stories, fables, and facts. That concept is only partly true. The Bible has been looked upon as a book of history or as a record of ancient civilizations. But it only partly fulfills these criteria.

The Bible tells of God, it contains literary works of great wealth, and research has established its claims for historicity. But the theme of the Bible is, in reality, man and his relationship with God. God enters the Bible because of Deity's involvement with mankind. The Bible's literature is the work of man, and its history the reflection of man's walk through the ages.

So it is that the Bible is not a medical text. But it is a book containing vast stores of medical fact, history, and drama. Medicine has always been an avenue through which man has tried to deal with his beginnings, his physical handicaps and illnesses, and his inevitable fate. And the Bible is as full of medicine as it is of honest expressions of the physical conditions of the people it pictures.

Genesis, the book of beginnings, introduces the biblical record. "In the beginning God created the heaven and the earth,"[1] states Scripture without apology or equivocation. The Creation story thereupon explains the formulation of an ecological system with man as the central catalyst. Man was instructed to propagate so as to share the earth's bounty. But it was also mankind's duty to nurture his planet and to administer its resources according to the dictates of law. Disregard for natural law would bring disastrous consequences:

> . . . accursed shall be the ground on your account.
> With labour you shall win your food from it
> all the days of your life.
> It will grow thorns and thistles for you,
> none but wild plants for you to eat.
> You shall gain your bread by the sweat of your brow
> until you return to the ground;
> for from it you were taken.
> Dust you are, to dust you shall return.[2]

This naturalistic attitude was not without other explanations for the rapid appearance of ecological disintegration—including sickness—following the sin of Adam and Eve in the Garden of Eden. The biblical story is also theistic, and the people of the Bible recognized God as a direct force in their lives. ". . . I the Lord am your healer,"[3] Israel was once informed.

But to persons who became so aware of the presence of God in the process of healing came also the feeling that their omnipotent Benefactor was also the source of many calamities.

Though viewed with some skepticism by modern man, the Great Flood of Noah's day was very real to biblical peoples who lived in its shadow. Real also were the great disasters of uncontrolled epidemics and recurrent warfare. Wind, water, fire, good health, death, victory, defeat—whatever—God was given the blame or the credit.

Sometimes the Bible makes the explicit point that God had directed events to transpire to His people, such as in the Babylonian captivity of Judah. And though biblical peoples would look to Deity as the source of bad health, God took specific care to point out that there were rational explanations for the fact of sickness in the world.

". . . take my words to heart, and the years of your life shall be multiplied,"[4] God counseled. And in the health laws given by God through Moses was the conditional aspect—obey and enjoy good health—disobey and suffer illness. Well might God expect such results. For when modern medicine has examined the health laws given to the chosen people it has discovered profound medical logic dating back many hundreds of years into the past.

New Testament believers were made part of the same philosophy when they were told that "a man reaps what he sows."[5]

Also stressed throughout the Bible is the concept of man who stands in a particular relationship to God. It was through that relationship that faith was given significance in the healing process. Naaman's faith, weak as it was, led him to wash in the Jordan River and receive healing.[6] "Your faith has cured you,"[7] Christ assured the woman suffering from vaginal hemorrhage.

And finally, medicine in the Bible is apocalyptic with its

emphasis on the final triumph of healing over the afflictions of mankind. John the Revelator looked forward to that great moment when ". . . there shall be no more death, neither sorrow, nor crying, neither shall there be any more pain."[8]

This glimpse of what will be is the core of medicine and health laws as recorded in the Bible. Good health is the goal of modern medicine. To have studied medicine in the Bible is to have gained a glimpse of what is good in the strivings of mankind for ultimate and complete healing.

Scripture References for Introduction

1 Genesis 1:1 KJV
2 Genesis 3:17–19 NEB
3 Exodus 15:26 NEB
4 Proverbs 4:10 NEB
5 Galatians 6:7 NEB
6 2 Kings 5:1–14
7 Matthew 9:22 NEB
8 Revelation 21:4 KJV

The Bible Book of Medical Wisdom

1

BONE OF MY BONES

The First Surgery

Surgery as a medical specialty receives little recognition in the Bible. Circumcision is the one surgical procedure irrevocably given to the world through biblical peoples. Military surgery doubtless became fairly well developed during the many battles recorded in the Bible, but scant mention is made of it.

Surgical dressing was spoken of allegorically by Ezekiel who stated that God had "broken the arm of Pharaoh king of Egypt; and, lo, it shall not be bound up to be healed, to put a roller to bind it, to make it strong to hold the sword."[1]

In one sense surgery was widely practiced by the Jews as they prepared animals for various sacrifices. This at least gave potential for education in basic anatomy—a fact demonstrated in the many descriptions of organs made in conjunction with sacrifices.[2] But Jewish law prohibited intentional dissection of the dead. This kept God's people from some of the barbaric rituals involving human sacrifice such as were practiced by the heathen nations around them.

However, in the opening words of the biblical narrative is found one description of a surgical procedure so classic in technique and so compelling in its implications that it alone gives the Bible stature in the antiquity of surgery.

The biblical record of the creation of man is simple. Of

Adam's creation it is stated that "the Lord God formed a man from the dust of the ground and breathed into his nostrils the breath of life. Thus the man became a living creature."[3]

But God took note that: "It is not good for the man to be alone. I will provide a partner for him. . . . And so the Lord God put the man into a trance, and while he slept, he took one of his ribs and closed the flesh over the place. The Lord God then built up the rib, which he had taken out of the man, into a woman."[4]

The similarities between God's surgical removal of a rib from Adam and the same modern surgical procedure are striking:

THE BIBLICAL DESCRIPTION	THE MODERN PROCEDURE
The Lord God put the man into a trance	Preoperative sedation
And while he slept	General anesthetic
He took one of his ribs	Rib resection—the surgery
And closed the flesh over the place	Closing of the surgical incision

With the story of history's first surgery the saga of medicine in the Bible begins.

Scripture References for Chapter 1

1   Ezekiel 30:21 KJV
2   Leviticus 1:1–17
3   Genesis 2:7 NEB
4   Genesis 2:18, 21, 22 NEB

2

CIRCUMCISION

The Surgical Covenant

The origin of circumcision among the ancients remains unknown. The rite of excising the male foreskin is known to have been practiced among many early peoples. The Egyptians circumcised the priestly class and other select males. This is well established in Egyptian art.

Regardless of the origin of circumcision it is clear that God's command to Abraham and his progeny gave the rite its destiny. As such it was the predominant surgery of biblical times.

When Abraham was ninety years of age God came to him with the promise that he would be the "father of a host of nations."[1] This covenant was to be remembered by a unique ceremony to be observed through all time:

> . . . circumcise yourselves, every male among you. You shall circumcise the flesh of your foreskin, and it shall be the sign of the covenant between us. Every male among you in every generation shall be circumcised on the eighth day. . . .[2]

Circumcision was not practiced during Israel's forty years of wandering away from Egyptian bondage. When Joshua led Israel into the Promised Land God commanded that circumcision be done on all the males who had been born during the desert wanderings. At Gibeath-haaraloth (the Hill of Foreskins) flint knives were made and the nation was circumcised. Physically traumatic, the surgical procedure was enough to make the Israelites stay "until they had recovered."[3]

Following this, circumcision became an act of supreme significance within Judaism.

When aliens aligned themselves with the Jewish nation they were circumcised.[4] Even during times of persecution against the Jews circumcision was practiced and Jewish identity was maintained—often at risk of life.

The story of David's dowry is fitting folklore in the annals of circumcision. King Saul, hoping to place David in a battle where he would be killed, asked David for the foreskins of a hundred Philistines as dowry for Michal, Saul's daughter. "Before the appointed time, David went out with his men and slew two hundred Philistines; he brought their foreskins and counted them out to the king in order to be accepted as his son-in-law."[5]

As a Jew, Christ was circumcised when He was eight days old[6] as was John the Baptist.[7]

With the rise of Christianity a great debate over circumcision nearly split the Church. A group of Jewish Christians insisted that Gentiles joining the Church needed circumcision to guarantee salvation. This and other questions were resolved in the first general conference of the Church which was held in Jerusalem. It was decided that circumcision was not needed and that the Church should "impose no irksome restrictions on those of the Gentiles who are turning to God."[8] Though this decision was supported by Paul, he later circumcised Timothy "out of consideration for the Jews."[9] Timothy's mother was Jewish, his father a Gentile.

Circumcision has had great medical significance if for no other reason than the millions of times the surgery has been performed.

No record is made in the Bible of the male infants who bled

to death following circumcision, although this undoubtedly occurred.

One simple aspect of God's command to Abraham helped prevent excessive bleeding with circumcision of the newborn. That was the instruction that the rite should be done on the eighth day of life. Modern medicine has come to understand the mechanisms at work in the clotting of blood. Of major importance in blood clotting is prothrombin, a compound made in the liver and the precursor of the active clotting agent thrombin. It has been well established that within a few hours after birth prothrombin becomes relatively depleted and does not become replenished by the infant's liver until about the eighth day of life.

Circumcision was a useful adjunct to hygiene, especially for nomadic peoples such as the early Israelites. Not only did it diminish the occurrence and severity of balanitis (inflammation of the penis), but it possibly helped control the spread of venereal diseases such as *Trichomonas vaginalis.*

Related to the poorer hygiene in some uncircumcised males is the increased incidence of cancer of the penis in this group. Very few cases of penile cancer have been found in circumcised males.

Of even more significance is the epidemiological relationship noted between cancer of the uterine cervix and circumcision of the male sexual partner. Many investigators have observed the low incidence of cervical cancer in Jewish women. The high incidence of cervical cancer in women whose sexual partners have not been circumcised probably comes from the transmission of a virus or other cancer-inducing agent from the male during coitus.

A surgical procedure in close anatomical relationship to circumcision is castration. Castration was widely practiced by the ancients, especially upon the courtiers of royalty.

Men who had either been surgically or accidently castrated were excluded from the congregation of the Lord.[10] This implies that castration was not practiced by the Jews. But the Bible makes eunuchs a matter of record in many places[11] including Christ's observation that "there are some eunuchs, which were so born from their mother's womb: and there are some eunuchs, which were made eunuchs of men: and there be eunuchs, which have made themselves eunuchs. . . ."[12] In this passage Christ not only mentioned surgical castration, but spoke of men lacking testicles "from their mother's womb." This statement could allude to either males with undescended testicles or to males suffering from certain congenital anomalies.

Scripture References for Chapter 2

1   Genesis 17:6 NEB
2   Genesis 17:10–12 NEB
3   Joshua 5:8 NEB
4   Genesis 34:14–17; Exodus 12:48
5   1 Samuel 18:27 NEB
6   Luke 2:21
7   Luke 1:59
8   Acts 15:20 NEB
9   Acts 16:3 NEB
10   Deuteronomy 23:1
11   Genesis 37:36
    1 Chronicles 28:1
    Jeremiah 29:2
    Acts 8:27–39
12   Matthew 19:12 KJV

3

THE EXODUS

The Egyptian Plagues

Along the Nile River nature has often played cruel games against people who through the centuries have deified its greatness and lived off its bounty. The ancient Egyptians found in the Nile fish and fowl, water for navigation and irrigation, and along its banks sites for eternal monuments.

To the Egyptians of the delta and to the Hebrew slaves of the kingdom, the Nile was the river which gave up Moses— first as an adopted member of Egypt's royalty, then as God's mighty deliverer of His people. After God had confronted him in the burning bush of the wilderness sanctuary, Moses turned back to his people enslaved along the Nile. And to the river where he had floated as a babe in a rush basket, Moses returned to call forth the plagues sent by the God of Abraham, Isaac, and Jacob.

Through Moses the great Jehovah's words to Pharaoh were plain: "Let my people go."[1] When Pharaoh disclaimed knowledge of this Hebrew Deity, God proclaimed:

Then will I show sign after sign and portent after portent in the land of Egypt. When I put forth my power against the Egyptians and bring the Israelites out from them, then Egypt will know that I am the Lord.[2]

Pharaoh refused to release the Hebrews and Moses struck the waters of the Nile with his staff. The once pure waters turned red like blood.[3] In quick and devastating succession other plagues followed. Frogs swarmed from the polluted Nile, died, and were piled into "countless heaps" until the "land stank."[4] Maggots[5] bred among the dead frogs only to turn into the "dense swarms of flies"[6] which brought disease to the cattle of the land[7] and boils[8] upon man and animals.

As Pharaoh became more obstinate God sent lightning and hail from the heavens which "beat down every growing thing and shattered every tree."[9] Locusts[10] and darkness[11] followed, blown upon the land by the hot desert winds. Then in a mighty display of power God struck dead the first-born of the Egyptians: "the first-born of Pharaoh who sits on his throne, the first-born of the slave-girl at the handmill, and all the first-born of the cattle."[12] When the night of anguish was over the Egyptians begged the Hebrews to leave. The Exodus began towards Canaan.

Medicine sees in the plagues of Egypt a sequence of occurrences which are related to epidemics. Microorganisms of the *Gymnodinium* species cause "red tides" polluting water and killing waterlife. Diseased amphibians like frogs swarm to land, die, and become the food for disease-transmitting insects. The death of animals and man soon follows in unprotected populations.

The Egyptians and Hebrews of the Exodus rightfully attributed to God's power in nature the source of the plagues. But from a medical viewpoint God was not as evident in the devastation of Egypt as in the preservation of the Hebrews and their animals from the mortal disasters and epidemics.

As the Hebrews left Rameses—their 430 years' sojourn in Egypt over—they had ample evidence that the great I Am[13] was indeed leading them to their Promised Land.

Scripture References for Chapter 3

1   Exodus 5:1 NEB
2   Exodus 7:3,5 NEB
3   Exodus 7:17
4   Exodus 8:15 NEB
5   Exodus 8:17
6   Exodus 8:24 NEB
7   Exodus 9:2–7
8   Exodus 9:8–12
9   Exodus 9:25 NEB
10 Exodus 10:12–20
11 Exodus 10:21–23
12 Exodus 11:5 NEB
13 Exodus 3:14

4

A MEDICAL PLAN FOR ISRAEL

The Mosaic Health Laws

In the milieu of antiquity disease, injury, and death were the common heritage of mankind. Egyptian and Babylonian medicine, with its description of the all-pervasive diseases suffered by the ancients, has been well described. Burial grounds from these and other ancient civilizations have yielded not only written descriptions of man's afflictions, but skeletons and mummified remains bearing mute evidence of the disease processes which brought people to early and agonizing deaths.

Intermixed among the incriminating evidence of the diseases afflicting the ancients have been found their pathetic attempts at understanding disease processes and treating those persons so afflicted. In both Babylonian and Egyptian medicine, healing was based upon ritualistic and mystical incantations little related to good treatment and often detrimental to the patient. In systems of healing where models of sheep's livers were examined for prognostic signs and animal dung served as balm for open wounds, little could be expected by the sick except that mystical existence beyond life to which physicians hastened their transport.

And in the pantheistic and polytheistic structure of most ancient civilizations the priest-healers cemented their errors of treatment with the authority of their office.

The Israelites in Egypt could not hope to escape their medical dilemma as they lived in abject servitude. Only in God was there to be hope. And in the help which came to them from God was not only their healing, but a system of health laws so remarkable as to seem modernistic in this age of advance.

The biblical record makes plain God's plan and how He carried it out. Scripture presents Him as the direct force in leading Israel out of its bondage in Egypt to the solitude of a wilderness where He would heal His people and give them a code of healthful living. But healing and health depended upon obedience. In the wilds of Shur came God's challenge to His people:

> If only you will obey the Lord your God, if you will do what is right in his eyes, if you will listen to his commands and keep all his statutes, then I will never bring upon you any of the sufferings which I brought on the Egyptians; for I the Lord am your healer.[1]

Conditioned upon the Israelite's faithfulness, God promised to make them the "head" and not the "tail."[2]

But if the people were to reject the health laws given to them retribution in the form of sickness was promised:

> . . . the Lord will strike you and your descendants with unimaginable plagues, malignant and persistent, and with sickness, persistent and severe. He will bring upon you once again all the diseases of Egypt which you dread, and they will cling to you. The Lord will bring upon you sickness and plague of every kind not written down in this book of the law, until you are destroyed.[3]

Although Israel was a theocracy, its health was not to be based on merely the observance of religious laws, but laws which claimed to be medical in nature. And the priests would be the wardens of the health laws—not in a position of religious magicians, but as leaders of the community.

As the health laws given to ancient Israel are studied in the light of modern medicine their inherent genius becomes apparent. With the superstition, false logic, and unsound principles upon which medicine was based until the past two centuries (and less) of human existence, it appears that neither Moses nor a consortium of consultants could have conjured the Levitical health laws without also contributing nonsensical regulations common in primitive medicine.

A typical public health law with great scientific merit governed housing which appeared unfit for human occupancy. According to this law if an area in a house developed a fungus infestation the house was declared unfit for habitation for seven days. If, at the end of the seven days, the mold remained, it was to be scraped from its location in the house. Fresh building materials were to be placed in the area of fungal growth. If the growth returned, the house was to be dismantled, "stones, timber, and daub, and it shall all be taken away outside the city to an unclean place."[4] The genius of this law is the probability that a house which developed fungal growth was apparently built in such a location or in such a fashion to be a good breeding area for not only fungus, but mosquitos and other insects which would be disease vectors.

The laws diagnosing and quarantining skin diseases like leprosy guaranteed that infectious diseases would not be spread with abandon throughout Israel.[5]

In a similar fashion the bodies of dead humans, animals, and insects were considered contaminated and strict laws governed the handling of these potentially infective objects.[6] The fastidious bathing requirements attached to these laws were of profound significance in the control of disease.

Infectious diseases which caused discharges were considered particularly dangerous and persons or animals with these discharges were isolated from other people. Whatever the discharge touched was either effectively cleansed or destroyed.[7] This helped limit the spread of tuberculosis, venereal diseases, and many bacterial and parasitic infections.

The common spread of diseases caused by the fecal contamination of drinking water and food was to be controlled with the first rational waste disposal law: "You shall have a sign outside the camp showing where you can withdraw. With your equipment you will have a trowel, and when you squat outside, you shall scrape a hole with it and then turn and cover your excrement."[8] Not only did this place human body waste outside the camp, but its burial at a shallow depth assured its quick decomposition by microorganisms in the ground. Blood, an attracter of disease-bearing insects and a culture medium for bacteria, was also to be buried.[9]

Adultery, sexual perversions, consanguineous marriages, and divorce were strictly proscribed with laws preventing the spread of venereal diseases, the inbreeding of genetic defects, and antisocial activities.[10] Laws governing childbirth and sexual intercourse protected women from pelvic infections and assured fertility.[11]

Dietary laws prohibited the eating of scavengers which would be likely vectors of infectious diseases.[12] Similar laws forbade the eating of animals which had died from disease or been attacked by other animals.[13] Blood and fat could not be eaten.[14] Especially did this mitigate against early development of heart attacks and strokes.

In one of Judaism's great contributions to mankind, a weekly Sabbath was made mandatory, providing for physical and mental rest and for spiritual refreshing. Coupled with this law —one of the Ten Commandments—was the admonition to fill the other six days of the week with physical work.[15] This, in itself, is a health law of significance.

Laws governing the well-being of animals and the cultivation of crops indirectly proved physically beneficial by making both more productive for the Israelites. Animals of different species were not to be mated.[16] Two different crops were not to be planted in the same field.[17] Every seventh year the land was to remain idle to prevent depletion of the soil.[18] And every fiftieth year large landholdings were to be broken up to assure that all persons would have land to cultivate.[19]

Medical jurisprudence was well developed in the Levitical laws. Many persons have viewed the law which allowed the taking of an "eye for eye" or a "hand for hand"[20] as being severely retributive. However, in the light of persons who were capable of committing murder for a lesser injury, this law seems to have protected the wrongdoer to some extent.

Murder was prohibited[21] but killing in defense was allowed, as evidenced in the permission to wage certain wars. Capital punishment was meted out for murder.[22] But to protect a person who was wrongly accused of murder, cities of refuge were designated to which the accused person could flee and be assured of a fair trial.[23]

Injury which was accidently inflicted upon a person was to be paid for in what was the first workmen's compensation insurance.

> When men quarrel and one hits another with a stone or with a spade, and the man is not killed but takes to his bed; if he recovers so as to walk about outside with a stick, then the one who struck him has no liability, except that he shall pay for loss of time and shall see that he is cured.[24]

If a woman was caused to miscarry because of injury, compensation was to be made for her injury.[25]

Injuries inflicted by animals were to be paid for by the owner of the animal. This included injuries to humans or other animals.[26] Compensation was likewise to be given when animals were injured by man or his carelessness.[27]

The poor were to be protected from starvation by being able to glean crops from the excess in the fields.[28]

The handicapped were protected. "You shall not treat the deaf with contempt," God told the Israelites, "nor put an obstruction in the way of the blind."[29]

In all this and more God's people were designed to rise above the ravages of sickness, poverty, and social ills. They were to be an example to the surrounding nations of the wisdom, love, and power of God. With God as Israel's healer the prophecy of Zechariah was the wished-for ideal:

> These are the words of the Lord of Hosts: Nations and dwellers in great cities shall yet come; people of one city shall come to those of another and say, 'Let us go and entreat the favour of the Lord, and resort to the Lord of Hosts; and I will come too.' So great nations and mighty peoples shall resort to the Lord of Hosts in Jerusalem and entreat his favour. These are the words of the Lord of Hosts. In those days, when ten men from nations of every language pluck up courage, they shall pluck the robe of a Jew and say, 'We will go with you because we have heard that God is with you.'[30]

Scripture References for Chapter 4

1   Exodus 15:26 NEB
2   Deuteronomy 28:12 NEB
3   Deuteronomy 28:59–61 NEB
4   Leviticus 14:45 NEB
5   Leviticus 13, 14
6   Numbers 19:11,12; Leviticus 11:27–40.
7   Leviticus 15:1–4.
8   Deuteronomy 23:12,13 NEB
9   Leviticus 17:13
10   *See* Chapter 14
11   *See* Chapter 15
12   Leviticus 11; Deuteronomy 14

13 Deuteronomy 14:21; Leviticus 22:8
14 Leviticus 7:24–27
15 Exodus 20:8–11
16 Leviticus 19:19
17 Leviticus 19:19
18 Leviticus 25:1–7
19 Leviticus 25:8–22
20 Exodus 21:23–25
21 Exodus 20:13; Numbers 35:9–34
22 Exodus 21:12
23 Exodus 21:13,14
24 Exodus 21:18,19
25 Exodus 21:22
26 Exodus 21:28–32; 35, 36
27 Exodus 21:33–34
28 Leviticus 19:9,10
29 Leviticus 19:14
30 Zechariah 8:20–23 NEB

5

OLD TESTAMENT MEDICINE

An Overview

Literature bears its own credentials. It is true that the Bible claims to bear messages about God and His dealings with men. But in addition to this the Bible claims to have wrapped those expressions in the voices and writings of real human beings. Many centuries of human expression—not only about God, but about everyday experiences—unite mankind in a common bond. These experiences include birth and death, illness and health. Medically, the Bible is not fiction, for when the medical problems of its people were written, the descriptions were too real, too exact. Medically, the Bible bears its own credentials.

Trauma is as real to everyone as a cut finger or a broken arm. It can happen by accident, be self-inflicted as in suicide, or it can be the result of murder or war. Trauma happened to biblical people.

Abimilech was such an unfortunate person. He was leading his forces against a defended tower in the city of Thebez when "a woman threw a millstone down on his head and fractured his skull. He called hurriedly to his young armour-bearer and said, 'Draw your sword and dispatch me, or men will say of me: A woman killed him.' So the young man ran him through and he died."[1]

Another severe head injury resulted in the death of the

Canaanite general, Sisera, during the time of the judges in ancient Israel. Routed in battle, Sisera ran on foot from the scene. He stopped for rest and food in what he felt was a friendly settlement. Mistaken, he fell into the hands of Jael. Seeing her advantage, Jael "took a tent-peg, picked up a hammer, crept up to him, and drove the peg into his skull as he lay sound asleep. His brains oozed out on the ground, his limbs twitched, and he died."[2] It is significant that the writer of Judges described accurately Sisera's neurological response to the fatal blow to his head.

Sisera was not the only enemy of Israel to suffer fatal brain damage in wars against God's people. Goliath literally lost his head in the ever famous fight with the young David.

Giants—along with other unusual variations of human size or form—have always awed people consigned to normality. Goliath was one of those awesome sights to the frightened soldiers of Israel as they squared off against the Philistines at Socoh. Undoubtably Goliath suffered from a dysfunction of the anterior pituitary gland which causes an increased secretion of growth hormone.

As in the case of Goliath, if excess growth hormone is secreted before the epiphyses close, gigantism results. Goliath had not only very great stature but also enough associated facial deformity to indeed make him a fearsome sight to Israel.

The New English Bible states that Goliath "was over nine feet in height."[3] David was brave in fighting Goliath. In actuality, however, David probably had the advantage over Goliath. The giant—dressed in his heavy armor—was awkward of movement and slow in response. The fleet-footed shepherd boy of Israel had little difficulty in approaching the stumbling giant. This, of course, takes nothing away from David in his great victory for Israel:

> When the Philistine began moving towards him again, David ran quickly to engage him. He put his hand into his bag, took out a stone, slung it, and struck the Philistine on the forehead.

The stone sank into his forehead, and he fell flat on his face on the ground. So David proved the victor with his sling and stone; he struck Goliath down and gave him a mortal wound, though he had no sword. Then he ran to the Philistine and stood over him, and grasping his sword, he drew it out of the scabbard, dispatched him and cut off his head.[4]

Goliath was not the only giant which Israel had fought and conquered during its many wars. During their wanderings in the wilderness following the exodus from Egypt the Israelites were forced to battle with Og, king of Bashan. Og was a giant, though his exact height is not given. His bedstead, however, "was nearly fourteen feet long and six feet wide."[5]

It was not uncommon for military loss to be followed by physical maiming of some of the leaders of the captured people. Following this practice Nebuchadnezzar, king of Babylon, put out the eyes of Judah's king Zedekiah at the fall of Jerusalem in 587 B.C.[6] This was the same fate suffered by Samson at the hands of the Philistines.[7]

When Israel defeated Adoni-bezek, a ruler of one of the Palestinian tribes, "they took him prisoner and cut off his thumbs and his great toes."[8] Adoni-bezek acknowledged this as just retribution as he had once done the same thing to seventy of his political enemies.

One enemy of Israel would have had just the right amount of fingers and toes if he had had his thumbs and great toes amputated. This man suffered from polydactyly, a congenital anomaly in which a person develops more than a normal number of digits. The particular man was a relative of Goliath, was also a giant, and had "six fingers on each hand and six toes on each foot, twenty-four in all."[9]

Left-handedness is mentioned at least twice in the Old Testament. Ehud was the Benjamite who murdered the king of Moab as Israel fought that heathen tribe. This is an episode of biblical intrigue:

Ehud made himself a two-edged sword, only fifteen inches long, which he fastened on his right side under his clothes, and he brought the tribute to Eglon, king of Moab. Eglon was a very fat man. When Ehud had finished presenting the tribute, he sent on the men who had carried it, and he himself turned back from the Carved Stones at Gilgal. 'My lord king,' he said, 'I have a word for you in private.' Eglon called for silence and dismissed all his attendants. Ehud then came up to him as he sat in the roof-chamber of his summer palace and said, 'I have a word from God for you.' So Eglon rose from his seat, and Ehud reached with his left hand, drew the sword from his right side and drove it into his belly. The hilt went in after the blade and the fat closed over the blade; he did not draw the sword out but left it protruding behind. Ehud went out to the porch, shut the doors on him and fastened them. When he had gone away, Eglon's servants came and, finding the doors fastened, they said, 'He must be relieving himself in the closet of his summer palace.' They waited until they were ashamed to delay any longer, and still he did not open the doors of the roof-chamber. So they took the key and opened the doors; and there was their master lying on the floor dead. While they had been waiting, Ehud made his escape.[10]

Another remarkable record of left-handedness is the instance of seven hundred warriors of Gibeah who were left-handed and "who could sling a stone and not miss by a hair's breadth."[11]

Orthopedic defects were among those keeping a man from the priesthood. Among defects listed were "a lame man, a man stunted or overgrown, a man deformed in foot or hand."[12]

Not all orthopedic problems were congenital or traumatic. King Asa of Judah is listed as one of those kings who followed God as he led the chosen people. When he got old, however, he did not leave his own fate in God's hand—to his great harm. "And Asa in the thirty and ninth year of his reign was diseased in his feet, until his disease was exceeding great: yet in his disease he sought not to the Lord, but to the physicians. And Asa slept with his fathers, and died."[13]

As Asa's feet problems came on in his old age, it could be surmised that he either developed arteriosclerotic gangrene, varicose veins with ulceration, or severe arthritis. Gout has also been suggested.

On the other hand Mephibosheth became traumatically crippled at the age of five years. During a time in history when physical handicaps provoked extreme hardship the story of Mephibosheth becomes unique.

Mephibosheth was the son of Jonathan, the son of King Saul and close friend of David. In the turbulent days of feudal fighting during Israel's early years as a kingdom, Saul and Jonathan were killed by the forces which soon made David king. Mephibosheth was part of that moment: "He was five years old when word of the death of Saul and Jonathan came from Jezreel. His nurse had picked him up and fled, but in her hurry to get away he fell and was crippled."[14]

There is no way of diagnosing with certainty the cause of Mephibosheth's lameness. It is doubtful that simple fractured legs of a five-year-old would result in permanent lameness. Bone healing at that age is very spontaneous and usually complete. Far more likely would have been damage to the spinal cord or brain damage from a blow to the head.

Scripture bears out the fact of David's close friendship to Jonathan. For out of deference to that friendship David returned to Mephibosheth Jonathan's and Saul's estates and made him a part of the royal court in Jerusalem. Mephibosheth "had his regular place at the king's table, crippled as he was in both feet."[15] Furthermore, Mephibosheth had one son, Mica, through whom the lineage of Saul was continued.[16]

Orthopedics finds only tangential bearing to the story of the ghastly murder of Queen Jezebel. She was thrown from an upper window of the dwelling in which she was hiding, "and some of her blood splashed on to the wall and the horses, which trampled her underfoot." In fulfillment of prophecy dogs then devoured her to an extent that when men went to bury Jezebel "they found nothing of her but the skull, the feet, and the palms of the hands."[17]

Couched in the symbolic language of Ezekiel is the "prophecy of the dry bones." God showed Ezekiel a large valley filled with bones. "They covered the plain, countless numbers of them, and they were very dry." Israel was in a period of spiritual apostasy—the people were dead and dried out in their relation to God. As a country Israel was also dried and separated like the bones. The ten northern tribes had been forever scattered in the destruction of Assyrian captivity more than one hundred years earlier. Now Judah was subjugated under Babylon's rule and was soon to go into complete captivity. Would there ever be hope of restoration—both spiritually and as a nation—for the chosen people? God's answer was the prophecy of the dry bones:

> 'This is the word of the Lord God to these bones: I will put breath into you, and you shall live. I will fasten sinews on you, bring flesh upon you, overlay you with skin, and put breath in you, and you shall live; and you shall know that I am the Lord.' . . . There was a rustling sound and the bones fitted themselves together. . . . breath came into them; they came to life and rose to their feet, a mighty host. . . . Prophesy, therefore, and say to them, These are the words of the Lord God: O my people, I will open your graves and bring you up from them, and restore you to the land of Israel. You shall know that I am the Lord when I open your graves and bring you up from them, O my people. Then I will put my spirit into you and you shall live, and I will settle you on your own soil, and you shall know that I the Lord have spoken and will act. . . .[18]

Lameness came to Jacob during a fateful night of wrestling with a stranger. Jacob was on his way to a reconciliation with Esau whom he had cheated out of a birthright some twenty years earlier. During a night of soul-searching and anguish, Jacob was suddenly attacked by a stranger. The terror-struck Jacob fought bitterly through the night. As daybreak came the mysterious assailant touched Jacob "in the hollow of his thigh, so that Jacob's hip was dislocated as they wrestled."[19]

Jacob then recognized that it was no mere mortal with whom he had been struggling. Even as his soul was wrestling in the anguish of his sin against Esau, so was Jacob thrown in a physical struggle with Deity. With such a realization Jacob pleaded for a blessing. The blessing was granted: "Your name shall no longer be Jacob, but Israel, because you strove with God and with men, and prevailed."[20]

The account confirms that Jacob's lameness came when he was struck "on that nerve in the hollow of the thigh."[21] This points plainly to a case of sciatica—pain, malfunction, and numbness—to the areas supplied by the sciatic nerve in the leg. A slipped intervertebral disc in the lower back would cause such symptoms as it pinched nerve roots making up the sciatic nerve.

Another neurological case history involved Nabal, an enemy of King David. Following a night of drunkenness, Nabal had "a seizure and lay there like a stone. Ten days later the Lord struck him again then he died."[22] Nabal had a cerebral vascular accident—a stroke. Following the initial attack Nabal lay comatose for ten days, then died.

A dramatic case of paralysis was that of the idolatrous King Jeroboam. A prophet bore the message from God that Josiah would be raised up to destroy idolatry in the land. King Jeroboam pointed at the prophet and commanded that he be seized. "Immediately the hand which he had pointed at him became paralyzed so that he could not draw it back."[23] Although this could have been nerve involvement, it is more likely that Jeroboam was struck with the psychiatric condition known as a conversion reaction or conversion hysteria. In conversion reaction the person suffers a motor function loss or sensory loss when his mind blocks out that neural unit. This could manifest itself as paralysis, blindness, or mutism. As could be expected, when the prophet prayed that Jeroboam's paralysis be removed, the king was healed. Such is often the suggestive nature of psychiatric disease.

There are three major cases of psychiatric illness recorded in the Old Testament. The first two were real, the third faked.

King Nebuchadnezzar brought Babylon to the pinnacle of its glory. Nebuchadnezzar was indeed a "king of kings." Under his despotism the entire civilized Middle East lived and gave him riches and glory. But because of his pride it was decreed by divine judgment that he would be humbled by mental illness until he realized "that the Most High is sovereign over the kingdom of men and gives it to whom he will."[24]

Refusing to heed the warning of the Prophet Daniel, Nebuchadnezzar went on his inevitable course towards disaster:

> All this befell King Nebuchadnezzar. At the end of twelve months the king was walking on the roof of the royal palace at Babylon, and he exclaimed, 'Is not this Babylon the great which I have built as a royal residence by my own mighty power and for the honor of my majesty?' The words were still on his lips, when a voice came down from heaven: 'To you, King Nebuchadnezzar, the word is spoken: the kingdom has passed from you. You are banished from the society of men and you shall live with the wild beasts; you shall feed on grass like oxen, and seven times will pass over you until you have learnt that the Most High is sovereign over the kingdom of men and gives it to whom he will.' At that very moment this judgement came upon Nebuchadnezzar. He was banished from the society of men and ate grass like oxen; his body was drenched by the dew of heaven, until his hair grew long like goats' hair and his nails like eagles' talons.

At the end of the appointed time, I, Nebuchadnezzar, raised my eyes to heaven and I returned to my right mind. I blessed the Most High, praising and glorifying the Ever-living One. . . .

At that very time I returned to my right mind and my majesty and royal splendor were restored to me for the glory of my kingdom.[25]

Nebuchadnezzar was suffering from either a manic-depressive or involutional psychosis. Specifically, he suffered from a rare condition, lycanthropy, wherein he felt he was, and acted like, an animal. Some have questioned the historicity of Nebuchadnezzar's illness because no records have been found of it in Babylonian sources. However, as most ancient dictator-kingships did not allow the chronicling of military or other defeats, this psychiatric embarrassment would understandably be left unmentioned.

Another biblical king who suffered severe psychiatric illness was Saul. Still shy and retiring as he was crowned to lead Israel, Saul soon came to know personal victory and defeat. Unable to stand up under criticism and the pressures of military challenges by the Philistines, Saul started to show signs of mental illness. Sensing this mental state the court servants secured David to play the harp to soothe Saul's nerves. This was effective "so that Saul found relief," until David became the heralded victor over the giant, Goliath.

Now furious with envy Saul once again requested David's harp music:

Next day an evil spirit from God seized upon Saul; he fell into a frenzy in the house, and David played the harp to him as he had before. Saul had his spear in his hand, and he hurled it at David, meaning to pin him to the wall; but twice David swerved aside. After this Saul was afraid of David, because he saw that the Lord had forsaken him and was with David.[26]

Saul's hatred and fear of David were complicated by continued military defeats at the hands of the Philistines. Behind this rose the specter of a deteriorating psychiatric illness. As defeat pressed in on him from every side, Saul finally made his way to the spiritualistic medium of Endor. This woman consorted with supposed spirits of the dead as she practiced her art—an art condemned by the death penalty in God's laws to Israel. Here Saul vainly sought an encouraging word from the spirit which purported to be the deceased prophet Samuel. Instead, defeat was predicted.[27]

A short while later Saul lay wounded in the battlefield. Unable to persuade his armor-bearer to kill him, Saul committed suicide.[28]

Saul showed signs of a manic-depressive personality. Periods of despondency gave way to acts of violence. He was also extremely paranoid when he thought of David's inevitable succession to the throne—a paranoia which led to Saul's attempted homicide of David.

David, Saul's great antagonist and eventual successor to Israel's throne, once had to fake insanity to protect his life. Fleeing from Saul, David found himself at Gath, a Philistine city. The people of Gath recognized David as the killer of thousands of Philistines—a point also noted by the king of Gath. Realizing his predicament David "became very much afraid of Achish, king of Gath. So he altered his behaviour in public and acted like a lunatic in front of them all, scrabbling on the double doors of the city gate and dribbling down his beard. Achish said to his servants, 'The man is mad! Why bring him to me? Am I short of madmen that you bring this one to plague me? Must I have this fellow in my house?'"[29]

Throwing his captors off guard by his actions, David made his escape.

Suicide, as committed by Saul, was apparently common during Old Testament times. Typical is the story of Ahithophel, an accomplice with Absalom in a plot against David. But as plots so often go, Ahithophel's turned sour.

When Ahithophel saw that his advice had not been taken he saddled his ass, went straight home to his own city, gave his last instructions to his household, and hanged himself.[30]

Diseases of the gastrointestinal tract were common during Old Testament times even though such maladies as diarrhea, hemorrhage, nausea, and vomiting gain scant mention. Vomiting is mentioned in connection with drunkenness.

A major bowel condition was suffered by King Joram (Jehoram) which terminated his reign and life. According to the biblical record Joram was an evil king who led the kingdom of Judah astray. Typical of the way the early Israelites looked upon disease the record is that "the Lord struck down the king with an incurable disease of the bowels. It continued for some time, and towards the end of the second year the disease caused his bowels to prolapse, and the painful ulceration brought on his death."[31] Joram was forty years of age when he died.

The case history points to Joram's disease as cancer of the rectum. The description is classic:

"Incurable disease"	The hopeless nature of cancer without treatment
"Continued for some time" (over two years)	The usual protracted nature of death by cancer
"Caused his bowels to prolapse"	The tumor's weight can cause its protrusion from the anus
"Painful"	Terminal cancer of the rectum would cause extreme pain without strong analgesics
"Ulceration"	The sloughing of dead tumor tissue brings about

this ulceration with its
bleeding and infection.

The case of Joram is the only definite description of cancer
in the entire Bible. It might have been less common then, but
many cases were probably impossible to diagnose by people
who were forbidden to do postmortem dissection.

One major problem suffered periodically throughout the
history of mankind was no stranger to biblical people. The
grim, stalking nature of starvation is classically described in
Lamentations:

> The sucking infant's tongue
>   cleaves to its palate from thirst;
> young children beg for bread
>   but no one offers them a crumb.
> Those who once fed delicately
>   are desolate in the streets,
> and those nurtured in purple
>   now grovel on dunghills.
> The punishment of my people is worse
>   than the penalty of Sodom,
> which was overthrown in a moment
>   and no one wrung his hands.
> Her crowned princes were once purer than snow,
>   whiter than milk;
> they were ruddier than branching coral,
>   and their limbs were lapis lazuli.
> But their faces turned blacker than soot,
>   and no one knew them in the streets;
> the skin was drawn tight over their bones,
>   dry as touchwood.
> Those who died by the sword were more fortunate
>   than those who died of hunger.[32]

Scripture References for Chapter 5

1 Judges 9:53,54 NEB
2 Judges 4:21, 22 NEB
3 1 Samuel 17:4 NEB
4 1 Samuel 17:48–51 NEB
5 Deuteronomy 3:11 NEB
6 2 Kings 25:7
7 Judges 16:21
8 Judges 1:6, 7 NEB
9 2 Samuel 21:20 NEB
10 Judges 3:16–26 NEB
11 Judges 20:16 NEB
12 Leviticus 21:19 NEB
13 2 Chronicles 16:12,13 KJV
14 2 Samuel 4:4 NEB
15 2 Samuel 9:13 NEB
16 2 Samuel 9:12
17 2 Kings 9:33,35 NEB
18 Ezekiel 37:5–14 NEB
19 Genesis 32:25 NEB
20 Genesis 32:28 NEB
21 Genesis 32:32 NEB
22 1 Samuel 25:37,38 NEB
23 1 Kings 13:4 NEB
24 Daniel 4:25 NEB
25 Daniel 4:28–34, 36 NEB
26 1 Samuel 18:10–12 NEB
27 1 Samuel 28
28 1 Samuel 31
29 1 Samuel 21:12–15 NEB
30 2 Samuel 17:23 NEB
31 2 Chronicles 21:18,19 NEB
32 Lamentations 4:4–9 NEB

6

OLD TESTAMENT MIRACLES

Elisha and Elijah

Although biblical miracles seem more prevalent in the New Testament, they are not absent in the writings of the Old Testament.

The healing of Naaman's leprosy is presented as having been miraculous. Naaman, the commander of the Syrian army under Ben-hadad II, king of Damascus, had become an unfortunate sufferer from leprosy. On one of many military campaigns which he led Naaman took captive a young Israelite girl. The girl was made a servant to Naaman's wife. Faithful to her heritage, the servant girl told of the prophet Elisha who could heal Naaman.

Desperate for relief from the dread disease Naaman arranged through Syria's king to travel to Samaria, the capital city of Israel. Naaman arrived in Samaria and presented Israel's king with a letter from king Ben-haded II. "This letter is to inform you that I am sending to you my servant Naaman, and I beg you to rid him of his disease."[1] Israel's horrified king interpreted this request as an excuse for Syria to make war. But Elisha recognized the opportunity such a healing would present to demonstrate the working of God in Israel.

Elisha's handling of Naaman seems unusual in the average physician-patient relationship. Elisha never went to meet Naaman. Instead, a message was sent to the Syrian commander that he was to bathe seven times in the River Jordan. Naaman was furious: "I thought he would at least have come out and stood, and invoked the Lord his God by name, waved his hand over the place and so rid me of the disease. Are not Abana and Pharpar, rivers of Damascus, better than all the waters of Israel? Can I not wash in them and be clean?"[2]

Restrained by his servants, Naaman finally acquiesced to Elisha's prescription for healing, "And his flesh was restored as a little child's, and he was clean."[3]

Naaman—joyous and thankful—returned to Elisha with offers of gold, silver, and expensive clothing. Elisha refused the gifts, accepting only from Naaman the Syrian's expression of conversion to the God of Israel.

Gehazi, a servant of Elisha, was confounded at the prophet for passing up such wealth. Gehazi lied to Naaman and received a gift from the homeward-bound Syrian. Elisha knew of his servant's deception. Confronting Gehazi with the fraudulently obtained wealth, Elisha predicted: "You may buy gardens with it, and olive-trees and vineyards, sheep and oxen, slaves and slave-girls; but the disease of Naaman will fasten on you and on your descendants for ever."[4]

Possibly contracting the disease from the gifts he received from Naaman, Gehazi became a leper and an outcast in Israel.

Another miraculous healing which turned to eventual ashes was that of Hezekiah, the thirteenth king of Judah. Hezekiah, at about the time King Sennacherib of Assyria invaded Judah, neared death from a "boil." This was likely an abscess such as can be caused by tuberculosis. Having pleaded to God, Hezekiah was informed by the prophet Isaiah that he would be healed and would live for fifteen more years. Following instructions Hezekiah applied a "fig-plaster" to the abscess, and was healed.[5]

As a sign of healing God made the sun's light move back "ten steps"[6] on the sundial. As avid astronomers this spectacle in the heavens was not missed by the Babylonians of Mesopotamia. Sending an envoy to congratulate Hezekiah, Babylon's king Merodach-baladan learned of the great treasures of Jerusalem. Not forgotten, these treasures became Babylon's when that empire under Nebuchadnezzar overthrew Jerusalem.

Two restorations of life made medical history in the Old Testament. In the first case Elijah healed the son of the widow of Zarephath. The child had become progressively ill "until at last his breathing ceased."[7] Taking the boy to his room Elijah "breathed deeply upon the child three times and called on the Lord."[8] The boy was brought back to life.

A similar situation prevailed when the prophet Elisha was called to the bed where a Shunammite boy lay dead. The boy had died after a headache struck him as he worked under the blazing Palestinian sun.

Elisha prayed to the Lord concerning the dead child:

> Then getting on to the bed, he lay upon the child, put his mouth to the child's mouth, his eyes to his eyes and his hands to his hands; and, as he pressed upon him, the child's body grew warm. Elisha got up and walked once up and down the room; then, getting on to the bed again, he pressed upon him and breathed into him seven times; and the boy opened his eyes.[9]

What attracts modern medicine to these two miraculous restorations of life is the classic description of the fundamentals of mouth-to-mouth resuscitation. Particularly was the Shunammite's son subjected to this procedure of forced ventilation. Also apparent are the pressing movements which Elisha made on the child—simulating the current practice of closed-chest cardiac massage.

However, even if Elijah or Elisha utilized this mode of resuscitation the two healings were miraculous. For the treatment started long after the two children had died. Cardiopulmonary resuscitation has to be initiated within five to seven minutes following cessation of respiration and circulation in order to prevent irreversible damage to the brain.

Scripture References for Chapter 6

1   2 Kings 5:6 NEB
2   2 Kings 5:11, 12 NEB
3   2 Kings 5:14 NEB
4   2 Kings 5:26, 27 NEB
5   2 Kings 20:7 NEB
6   2 Kings 20:9–11 NEB
7   1 Kings 17:17 NEB
8   1 Kings 17:21 NEB
9   2 Kings 4:34, 35 NEB

7

SKIN AND FLESH, BONES AND SINEWS

Anatomy

Biblical peoples were well advanced in their knowledge of anatomy even though they were restricted in actual dissection of the human body.

It would be natural for the Hebrews to be aware of the body and its functions for their theistic viewpoint held God to be the Creator of the body and the Sustainer of life. It was God who formed "man from the dust of the ground and breathed into his nostrils the breath of life."[1]

Paul reiterated this Jewish concept to the Corinthian converts of New Testament times when he reminded them they were "God's temple, where the Spirit of God dwells."[2]

Limiting anatomical study of corpses were the Levitical laws prohibiting contact with the dead. "Whoever touches a corpse shall be ritually unclean for seven days."[3] Following contact with the dead a purification rite was required. Failure to perform this rite meant loss of citizenship.

The Israelites were also prohibited from offering human sacrifices as was the custom of human tribes surrounding them.[4]

Despite these restrictions the Bible confirms that the Hebrews astutely observed surface anatomy of the human body. War wounds were plenteous and allowed some investigation of internal organs. Skeletons of men and animals provided adequate material for studying bones. And the dissection of animals as part of the sacrificial rituals lent depth to anatomical knowledge.

To the ancient Hebrews the body was a whole comprised of interacting parts. Paul envisioned the "single body with its many limbs and organs, which, many as they are, together make up one body."[5]

Job queried God; "Didst thou not clothe me with skin and flesh and knit me together with bones and sinews?"[6]

Of the many citations of anatomical parts in the Bible, the following are prominent:

BLOOD: Blood was considered to be the life essence: "For the life of the flesh is in the blood."[7] Blood became a prominent symbol in the sin sacrifices. Loss of blood was equated with death.[8] Solomon in his wisdom noted that for those persons who were "churlish and arrogant wringing the nose produces blood."[9] Following Christ's death on the cross a Roman soldier pierced His side with a spear producing a flow of "blood and water."[10] This possibly represented the separation of Christ's blood into its two main parts—cells and serum—or it could have been blood and peritoneal fluid. Christians view the shedding of Christ's blood as the ultimate proof of His salvation effort for mankind.

BONES: Incomparable is the story of Ezekiel's vision of the valley filled with dry bones, where upon the command of God "there was a rustling sound and the bones fitted themselves together."[11] Bones were known to contain marrow[12] which could become infected and drain.[13] Deformed bones or joints excluded men from the priesthood.[14] Fractures[15] and dislocations[16] of bones were common among the ancients and difficult to treat. Goliath[17] had bones which were too long, and Zaccheus was a dwarf.[18]

SKIN AND HAIR: Skin covers the external surface of the body[19] giving protection from disease and allowing for the controlled loss of fluids and wastes through sweat. Skin diseases were endemic among the nomadic Hebrews, and the modernistic Levitical quarantine laws helped contain contagious skin problems.[20] Baldness was not considered a disease in man,[21] although the promiscuous women of Isaiah's day became bald—possibly from syphilis. When Elisha's baldness was mocked by children, bears came from the woods "and mauled forty-two of them."[22] White hair was recognized as a sign of old age,[23] and was to be respected: "You shall rise in the presence of grey hairs."[24] As a measure of God's concern for man's well-being, Christ assured His listeners that "even the hairs of your head have all been counted."[25]

BRAIN: Biblical writers evidently did not ascribe to the brain any of its higher motor or mental functions. One person who could have made this association was Jael. When she drove a tent peg into Sisera's skull "his brains oozed out on the ground, his limbs twitched, and he died."[26]

EYES: Blindness in the Bible is more completely discussed in chapter 23. Israel was as dear to God as "the apple of his eye,"[27] an apt synonym for the eyeball. God's omnipresence is portrayed in the Old Testament allegory: "The eyes of the Lord range through the whole earth."[28]

TEETH: Good teeth were a blessing to the ancients. Jacob's son, Judah, is said to have had "teeth whiter than milk."[29] Apparently in this phrase was noted the association between the drinking of milk and healthy teeth. So important were teeth that "tooth for tooth" retribution became part of the Levitical law.[30] In an unusual phraseology Job claimed to have escaped his torment by "the skin of my teeth."[31] Solomon lamented the diseased tooth in the couplet:

Like a tooth decayed or a foot limping
is a traitor relied on in the day of trouble.[32]

TONGUE: The tongue is necessary for correct speech. No description in the Bible of the power of speech and the tongue compares with that given by James:

What an immense stack of timber can be set ablaze by the tiniest spark! And the tongue is in effect a fire. It represents among our members the world with all its wickedness; it pollutes our whole being; it keeps the wheel of our existence red-hot, and its flames are fed by hell. Beasts and birds of every kind, creatures that crawl on the ground or swim in the sea, can be subdued and have been subdued by mankind; but no man can subdue the tongue. It is an intractable evil, charged with deadly venom. We use it to sing the praises of our Lord and Father, and we use it to invoke curses upon our fellow-men who are made in God's likeness.[33]

HEART: The heart was intimately associated with thought processes according to biblical writers. Man was to love God "with his whole heart";[34] that is with all his mental capacities. The anatomic location of the heart was noted when Joab killed Abner by stabbing him "under the fifth rib."[35] Heart disease was well described in Biblical times. Arteriosclerosis (hardening of the arteries) has been found in Egyptian mummies, and many have wondered if the "hardening" of Pharaoh's heart at the time of the Exodus did not refer to this condition.[36] It is more likely that he suffered from arteriosclerosis in the brain as shown by his stubbornness in freeing the Israelites. Job[37] and Jeremiah both suffered from heart palpitation. Jeremiah cried out, "Oh, the throbbing of my heart!"[38] As usual, Solomon's wisdom prevails even on the subject of the heart: "A merry heart makes a cheerful countenance."[39]

LIVER: The liver was known among the early Hebrews because of its dissection from sacrificial animals.[40] It and other internal organs of animals were burned on the altar. Babylonians in the days of Israel used models of the liver in their magical rites and medical incantations.

BOWELS: The close relationship between emotions and bowel function was not lost to biblical writers.[41] Jeremiah at times suffered from gas pains; "Oh, the writhing of my bowels."[42] Joram died from cancer of the rectum.[43] Judas was disemboweled while committing suicide.[44]

KIDNEYS AND ADRENAL GLANDS: The kidneys and adrenal glands were recognized by the Israelites in their sacrificial animals.[45] Described simply as the "fat" on the kidneys, the Levitical description of the adrenals is the only one coming from ancient medicine, Greek, Roman, or Arab. The functions of the kidneys or the adrenals were not known by the Israelites.

BREASTS: The female breasts have forever served as a source of sustenance and wonderment for mankind. Needless to say, their function as a food source was widely used by the ancients. So much was this the case that "dry breasts" were recognized as a major obstetrical calamity.[46] Showing great concern, the brothers in Solomon's Song lamented their sister's plight:

> We have a little sister
> who has no breasts;
> What shall we do for our sister
> when she is asked in marriage?[47]

As the smallest breasts can supply adequate milk for the newborn and large breasts do not insure good milk production, these brothers were evidently recognizing the sexual symbolism of breasts. This verity Solomon knew well. "My beloved is for me a bunch of myrrh as he lies on my breasts," sang the bride of Solomon's Song to the bridegroom.[48] "Your two breasts are like two fawns," responded the bridegroom.[49]

GENITALIA: Male genitalia are given earliest consideration in the Bible in the initiation of the rite of circumcision.[50] Through this ceremony alone the male foreskin was to achieve anatomical prominence throughout centuries. A severe deformity of the male external genitalia is mentioned in the assorted laws of Deuteronomy in reference to the man "whose testicles have been crushed or whose organ has been severed."[51] Male castration produced the eunuchs so frequently mentioned in the Bible.[52] The uterus is the location for fetal growth, a fact noted by David and other biblical writers.[53]

Scripture References for Chapter 7

1   Genesis 2:7
2   1 Corinthians 3:16 NEB
3   Numbers 19:14 NEB
4   Leviticus 18:21
5   1 Corinthians 12:12 NEB
6   Job 10:11 NEB
7   Leviticus 17:11 KJV
8   Genesis 9:6
9   Proverbs 30:32, 33 NEB
10 John 19:34 NEB
11 Ezekiel 37:7 NEB
12 Hebrews 4:12
13 Proverbs 12:4

14   Leviticus 21:19, 20
15   Ezekiel 30:21; Psalms 51:8
16   Genesis 32:25
17   1 Samuel 17:4
18   Luke 19: 2, 3
19   Ezekiel 37:8; Job 10:11
20   Leviticus 13
21   Leviticus 13:40, 41
22   2 Kings 2:24 NEB
23   Isaiah 46:4
24   Leviticus 19:32 NEB
25   Matthew 10:30 NEB
26   Judges 4:21 NEB
27   Deuteronomy 32:10 NEB
28   2 Chronicles 16:9 NEB
29   Genesis 49:12 NEB
30   Leviticus 24:20 NEB
31   Job 19:20 KJV
32   Proverbs 25:19 NEB
33   James 3:5–9 NEB
34   Luke 10:27
35   2 Samuel 3:27 KJV
36   Exodus 7:22 KJV
37   Job 37:1
38   Jeremiah 4:19 NEB
39   Proverbs 17:22 NEB
40   Leviticus 3:15
41   Philippians 1:8; 2:1 KJV
42   Jeremiah 4:19 NEB
43   2 Chronicles 21:18, 19
44   Acts 1:18
45   Leviticus 3:15
46   Hosea 9:14
47   Song of Solomon 8:8, 9 NEB
48   Song of Solomon 1:13 NEB

8

PLAGUE AND PESTILENCE

Epidemics

Until the advent of modern medicine, epidemics of disease played havoc with mankind. Indeed, whole nations were ruled by the whim of contagious disease. Epidemics often decimated populations or armies leaving them prey for more fortunate peoples.

Although God gave Israel remarkable public health laws designed to quarantine infectious disease and control its spread, the specter of epidemics is graphically portrayed in the Old Testament. The diseases described in the Old Testament are known to medicine, and periodically flare up to scourge unprotected populations of the modern world.

In the days when Isaiah was prophet in Israel and Hezekiah was king of that country, an Assyrian army approached Jerusalem. Nearing the peak of its power under Sennacherib, Assyria appeared capable of laying seige to Jerusalem and destroying Israel's capital. With prospects of national survival dim, Hezekiah turned to God for help. God's answer concerning the king of Assyria came through Isaiah:

> He shall not enter this city
> nor shoot an arrow there,
> he shall not advance against it with shield
> nor cast up a siege-ramp against it.

By the way on which he came he shall go back;
this city he shall not enter.
This is the very word of the Lord.
I will shield this city to deliver it,
for my own sake and for the sake of my servant David.[1]

Billeting near Jerusalem, Sennacherib's army readied for battle. "That night the angel of the Lord went out and struck down a hundred and eighty-five thousand men in the Assyrian camp; when morning dawned, they all lay dead."[2] Sennacherib was forced to retreat to Nineveh. This incident has been immortalized in Byron's "The Destruction of the Sennacherib."

The Assyrian came down like the wolf on the fold,
And his cohorts were gleaming in purple and gold;
And the sheen of their spears was like stars on the sea,
When the blue wave rolls nightly on deep Galilee.

Like the leaves of the forest when summer is green,
That host with their banners at sunset were seen:
Like the leaves of the forest when autumn hath blown,
That host on the morrow lay withered and strown.

For the angel of death spread his wings on the blast,
And breathed in the face of the foe as he passed;
And the eyes of the sleepers wax'd deadly and chill,
And their hearts but once heaved—and forever grew still.

And there lay the steed with his nostril all wide,
But through it there roll'd not the breath of his pride:
And the foam of his gasping lay white on the turf,
And cold as the spray of the rock beating surf.

And there lay the rider, distorted and pale,
With the dew on his brow and the rust on his mail;
And the tents were all silent, the banners alone,
The lances uplifted, the trumpet unblown.

And the widows of Ashur are loud in their wail,
And the idols are broke in the temple of Baal;
And the might of the Gentile, unsmote by the sword,
Hath melted like snow in the glance of the Lord!

LORD BYRON

God could easily have used natural disaster in the form of an epidemic as the cause of the Assyrian slaughter. Bubonic plague in its pneumonic form or cholera spread through drinking water are both capable of such devastation. The historian Herodotus attributed such a catastrophe to an infestation of field mice. This strongly implicates bubonic plague.

Bubonic plague in epidemic proportion has ravaged whole populations at various times throughout history. A classic description of an epidemic of bubonic plague is found in the Old Testament dating back to the days before Israel had its first king.

During military action against the Israelites the Philistines had captured the Ark of God—Israel's most sacred religious object. The Ark was taken to the city of Ashdod where it was placed in the temple of Dagon, the Philistinian fish-god. Calamity struck the Philistines; first when Dagon crashed to the floor in front of the Ark of God, and then when disease spread in the city.

Then the Lord laid a heavy hand upon the people of Ashdod; he threw them into distress and plagued them with tumours, and their territory swarmed with rats. There was death and destruction all through the city.[3]

Similar epidemics befell Gath and Ekron when the Ark was taken to those Philistinian cities. "There was death and destruction. Even those who did not die were plagued with tumours."[4]

Realizing that keeping the Ark of God would only bring more sickness and death the Philistines decided to send it back to Israel—but not without a gift of appeasement. The gift turned out to be gold models of five tumors and five rats.

The tumors from which the people suffered were swollen lymph nodes, the buboes of bubonic plague. The gold rats were apt testimony to the animal vector by which bubonic plague is spread. Fleas infested with *Pasteurella pestis* are carried by rats. When the rats die the fleas leave the body and infest humans. The fleabite transmits the microorganism to the human bloodstream, and bubonic plague results.

The Israelites did not escape diseases when they disobeyed the health laws given to them by God. One instance of rampant immorality during the exodus from Egypt resulted in a venereal-disease epidemic which ravaged the camp. The epidemic occurred following adultery with Moabite women. Twenty-four thousand persons are said to have died in this epidemic.[5]

On another occasion the Israelites—tired of the stringent diet during their desert wanderings—became gluttonous when a flock of quail was blown upon the camp. The meat had become infected in the desert heat causing the death of many Israelites from food poisoning.[6]

Scripture References for Chapter 8

1   2 Kings 19:32–34 NEB
2   2 Kings 19:35 NEB
3   1 Samuel 5:6 NEB
4   1 Samuel 5:11, 12 NEB
5   Numbers 25:1–9
6   Numbers 11

9

THE WAY OF A MAN WITH A MAID

Marriage and Sex

Three things there are which are too wonderful for me,
    four which I do not understand:
    the way of a vulture in the sky,
    the way of a serpent on the rock,
    the way of a ship out at sea,
    and the way of a man with a girl.[1]

In the Bible is found the claim for the origin of marriage. In the Genesis Creation story is portrayed the establishment of the marital unit which has continued as the basic structure of society to the present day. This was the first institution ordained by God and of its foundation it is stated; "It is not good for the man to be alone. I will provide a partner for him. The Lord God then built a woman. That is why a man leaves his father and mother and is united to his wife, and the two become one flesh."[2]

Marriage was designed to fill basic needs of mankind. Sexuality as such a need is not ignored in the marriage relationship as outlined in the Bible. The sexual side of marriage is directly implied in the Creation account in the observation that husband and wife "become one flesh."

For all that has been said about Paul and marriage it is clear that Paul recognized the sexual needs within the marital union. "The husband must give the wife what is due to her, and the wife equally must give the husband his due. The wife cannot claim her body as her own; it is her husband's. Equally, the husband cannot claim his body as his own; it is his wife's."[3]

Solomon knew well both the joys of marriage and the sorrows of adultery. Of the sexual relationship in marriage he counseled:

> Rejoice with the wife of thy youth. Let her be as the loving hind and pleasant roe; let her breasts satisfy thee at all times; and be thou ravished always with her love.[4]

The Song of Solomon remains a literary classic in its description of the beauty of marital and physical love. In portraying the attractions between man and woman this love song is summarized with the poetic call of the bridegroom to his select:

> Wear me as a seal upon your heart,
>   as a seal upon your arm;
> for love is strong as death,
> passion cruel as the grave;
>   it blazes up like blazing fire,
>   fiercer than any flame.
> Many waters cannot quench love,
>   no flood can sweep it away;
> if a man were to offer for love
>   the whole wealth of his house,
>   it would be utterly scorned.[5]

Solomon was not the only biblical writer to note the joys of marital love. Especially was the honeymoon period recognized as the time when a newly married couple should be free to enjoy each other. Such a right was this held to be that there was placed in the Mosaic code a honeymoon law: "When a man is newly married, he shall not be liable for military service or any other public duty. He shall remain at home exempt from service for one year and enjoy the wife he has taken."[6]

Not all biblical descriptions of love and sexuality assume the ascetic heights of the Song of Solomon. Biblical writers were not prudish about human sexuality. They wrote of people living real—and sometimes perverted—sexual lives.

Joseph in Egypt rejected the seductive proposition of Potiphar's wife by asking, "How can I do anything so wicked, and sin against God?"[7]

Not having such a strong will when tempted, King David saw the wife of Uriah, Bathsheba, openly bathing during a warm Palestinian evening. He lusted for her beauty, had intercourse with her, and impregnated her. To eliminate Uriah, David sent him into battle with instructions sent to the field commanders to make certain that Uriah would be killed. Upon Uriah's death David married Bathsheba.[8] David's sin became a curse to him, and in remorseful repentance he offered a prayer to God, "Create in me a clean heart, O God; and renew a right spirit within me."[9]

Brutal and ugly is the story of the men of Gibeah. Having failed in their attempt to homosexually assault a Levite visiting the town, they repeatedly raped his concubine until she died from the ordeal.[10]

Because of the sins of that city, Sodom[11] became synonymous with depraved sexual perversions. Israel's activities were at one time compared to Sodom by Isaiah.[12]

In an attempt to keep Israel from the sexual sins of the heathen nations surrounding them, God gave laws governing sexual activity. "You shall not commit adultery,"[13] God commanded from Mt. Sinai.

But far more explicit were other Levitical laws governing sexual relations. Transvestism, incest, or relations with near relatives were forbidden.[14] Homosexuality and bestiality were condemned: "You shall not lie with a man as with a woman: that is an abomination. You shall not have sexual intercourse with any beast to make yourself unclean with it, nor shall a woman submit herself to intercourse with a beast: that is a violation of nature."[15]

Paul in New Testament times cited homosexuality as a perverted passion of the Roman culture; "Women have exchanged natural intercourse for unnatural, and their men in turn, giving up natural relations with women, burn with lust for one another."[16]

Because of the story of Onan's sin[17] some have believed that masturbation is condemned in the Bible. (Actually, Onan's sin was his refusal to carry out patriarchical responsibilities with his brother's widow.) Levitical law apparently recognized male masturbation as a natural event, commanding only that "when a man has emitted semen, he shall bathe his whole body in water and be unclean till evening."[18]

Although sexual relations between unmarried people are strongly spoken against throughout the Bible, Levitical law did not punish the guilty with death as in cases of adultery or perversion. Instead, marriage was urged; "When a man seduces a virgin who is not yet betrothed, he shall pay the bride-price for her to be his wife."[19]

The Apostle Paul also knew of the strong attraction between the sexes. Regarding the girl friend Paul counseled the unmarried Corinthian male that if he "feels that he is not behaving properly towards her, if, that is, his instincts are too strong for him, and something must be done, let them marry."[20]

Although polygamous arrangements were common among the ancients, the Bible upholds monogamy as the marital ideal.

Divorce laws were given to the children of Israel.[21] But Christ made it plain that divorce should occur only in cases of adultery. "I tell you," Christ informed the questioning Pharisees, "if a man divorces his wife for any cause other than unchastity, and marries another, he commits adultery."[22]

The sexual life of man is very closely related to procreation. God commanded Adam and Eve to "be fruitful and increase, fill the earth."[23]

Because children came from marriage, infertility became looked upon as a curse. The fertile marriage was considered to be blessed by God. The psalmist made this poetically clear:

> Sons are a gift from the Lord
> and children a reward from him.
> Like arrows in the hand of a fighting man
> are the sons of a man's youth.
> Happy is the man
> Who has a quiver full of them.[24]

The relationships of husband, wife, and children toward each other are no better stated in Scripture than in Paul's comparison of the family unit with Christ's association with the Church.[25] Here husbands were told to love their wives, wives to respect their husbands, children to obey their parents, and fathers to instruct their children.

The responsibility of children to their parents made a part of the Ten Commandments. "Honor your father and your mother, that you may live long in the land which the Lord your God is giving you."[26]

As an exponent of monogamous marriage and as a polygamist by nature Solomon became an expert on the subjects of women, wives, lovers, and mothers. Certainly some of Solomon's wives made his life miserable. This is clear in the Proverbs he wrote:

> Like a gold ring in a pig's snout
> is a beautiful woman without good sense.[27]

> Better to live alone in the desert
> than with a nagging and ill-tempered wife.[28]

Endless dripping on a rainy day—
that is what a nagging wife is like.
As well try to control the wind as to control her!
As well try to pick up oil in one's fingers![29]

These verities should not be taken to mean that Solomon did not highly praise women and wives. Other Proverbs bear this out:

A capable wife is her husband's crown;
one who disgraces him is like rot in his bones.[30]

Home and wealth may come down from ancestors,
but an intelligent wife is a gift from the Lord.[31]

And unsurpassed is the description of the capable wife of Proverbs 31:

Who can find a capable wife?
Her worth is far beyond coral.
Her husband's whole trust is in her,
and children are not lacking.
She repays him with good, not evil,
all her life long.
She chooses wool and flax
and toils at her work.
Like a ship laden with merchandise,
she brings home food from far off.
She rises while it is still night
and sets meat before her household.
After careful thought she buys a field
and plants a vineyard out of her earnings.
She sets about her duties with vigor
and braces herself for the work.
She sees that her business goes well,

and never puts out her lamp at night.
She holds the distaff in her hand,
and her fingers grasp the spindle.
She is open-handed to the wretched
and generous to the poor.
She has no fear for her household when it snows,
for they are wrapped in two cloaks.
She makes her own coverings,
and clothing of fine linen and purple.
Her husband is well known in the city gate
when he takes his seat with the elders of the land.
She weaves linen and sells it,
and supplies merchants with their sashes.
She is clothed in dignity and power
and can afford to laugh at tomorrow.
When she opens her mouth, it is to speak wisely,
and loyalty is the theme of her teaching.
She keeps her eye on the doings of her household
and does not eat the bread of idleness.
Her sons with one accord call her happy;
her husband too, and he sings her praises:
'Many a woman shows how capable she is;
but you excel them all.'
Charm is a delusion and beauty fleeting;
it is the God-fearing woman who is honoured.
Extol her for the fruit of all her toil,
and let her labours bring her honour in the city gate.[32]

The Bible does not record that Christ ever married. But His attitudes towards marriage and sex are well preserved in the New Testament.

Christ recounted the creation of marriage in Eden by the union of man and woman. Then he added; "It follows that they are no longer two individuals: they are one flesh. What God has joined together, man must not separate."[33]

Christ's first miracle occurred at a wedding feast in the small town of Cana in Galilee. When the supply of wine became exhausted Christ replenished it at a request from His mother.[34]

Christ condemned adultery and extended the Levitical definition of the sin by proclaiming in the Sermon on the Mount: "If a man looks on a woman with a lustful eye, he has already commited adultery with her in his heart."[35]

Though Christ condemned adultery the great compassion of His ministry to mankind found no higher expression than in the cases of two adulterous women, the woman taken in adultery and the woman who loved much.

The Pharisees brought to Christ a woman caught in the act of adultery and demanded of Him if she should not be stoned to death in accordance with Levitical law. "That one of you who is faultless shall throw the first stone," Christ challenged the woman's tormentors. Conscience-stricken they fled leaving Christ alone with the accused. Assuring her that condemnation was not His purpose, Christ simply said, "You may go; do not sin again."[36]

Again, Christ was guest of honor at a banquet in a Pharisee's house when an immoral woman entered, opened a bottle of expensive perfume, and tearfully washed Christ's feet. The host was shocked at Christ letting such a woman attend Him. Turning to His host Christ said: "You see this woman? I came to your house: you provided no water for my feet; but this woman has made my feet wet with her tears and wiped them with her hair. You gave me no kiss; but she has been kissing my feet ever since I came in. You did not anoint my head with oil; but she has anointed my feet with myrrh. And so, I tell you, her great love proves that her many sins have been forgiven; where little has been forgiven, little love is shown."[37]

Christ knew the human mind. He knew the depths of sin. But He also knew of the power of forgiveness and the miracle of love. Love, said Christ, is the great commandment.[38]

Scripture References for Chapter 9

1   Proverbs 30:18, 19 NEB
2   Genesis 2:18, 22, 24 NEB
3   1 Corinthians 7:3, 4 NEB
4   Proverbs 5:18, 19 KJV
5   Song of Solomon 8:6, 7 NEB
6   Deuteronomy 24:5 NEB
7   Genesis 39:9 NEB
8   2 Samuel 11, 12
9   Psalms 51:10 KJV
10 Judges 19
11 Genesis 18, 19
12 Isaiah 1:4, 9, 10, 15, 20
13 Exodus 20:14 NEB
14 Leviticus 18:6–18; Deuteronomy 22:5
15 Leviticus 18:23 NEB
16 Romans 1:27 NEB
17 Genesis 38:2–10
18 Leviticus 15:16 NEB
19 Exodus 22:16 NEB
20 1 Corinthians 7:36 NEB
21 Deuteronomy 24:1–4
22 Matthew 19:9 NEB
23 Genesis 1:28 NEB
24 Psalms 127:3–5 NEB
25 Ephesians 4:22–5:4
26 Exodus 20:12 NEB
27 Proverbs 11:22 NEB
28 Proverbs 21:19 NEB
29 Proverbs 27:15, 16 NEB
30 Proverbs 12:4 NEB
31 Proverbs 19:14 NEB
32 Proverbs 31:10–31 NEB
33 Matthew 19:6 NEB

10

THE LAW OF JEALOUSY

Venereal Disease

To persons not medically oriented, the "Law of Jealousy," cited in Numbers 5, appears to be nothing more than superstitious religious ritual. The fault of that logic lies in taking a test which claims to be medical and not subjecting it to medical evaluation. Viewed from a medical standpoint, the Law of Jealousy becomes more than mysticism—it is a crude, but correct, method for diagnosing pelvic inflammatory disease. This is a symptom complex in women most commonly associated with gonorrhea, a venereal disease.

Though the Law of Jealousy would not make a correct diagnosis of pelvic inflammatory disease in every case (nothing in medicine is 100 percent) its high degree of right diagnoses would be guaranteed by one assumption. That assumption is that those women involved in extramarital sexual relations would likely have sexual contact with a carrier of a venereal disease. This would be a promiscuous person who was also without the benefit of modern antibiotics needed to cure venereal disease.

The Law of Jealousy allowed a man who was suspicious that his wife had been unfaithful to bring her before the priest for trial by ordeal. The trial consisted of the priest mixing temple water with dust and making the woman drink the "water of bitterness'' thus concocted. What followed was probably un-related to the "water of bitterness." It was the natural course of the pelvic infection which occurred in the guilty woman.

After the priest had made her drink the water:

> . . . if she be defiled, and have done trespass against her husband . . . the water that causeth the curse shall enter into her, and become bitter, and her belly shall swell, and her thigh shall rot: and the woman shall be a curse among her people. And if the woman be not defiled, but be clean; then she shall be free and shall conceive seed.[1]

The curse described is an outline of the main features of gonorrheal pelvic infection. As written, it could well be placed in a modern medical textbook. The main features of the curse and the disease can be enumerated.

1 *Bitterness:* Acutely ill women with pelvic infections are usually nauseated and vomit.

2 *Abdominal distension:* Peritonitis from the pelvic infec-tion causes poor intestinal function and accumulation of gas in the intestines. Also the severe pelvic and abdominal pain is not unlike that felt in actual abdominal distension.

3 *Thigh shall rot:* ("Miscarriage," NEB.) Acute pelvic inflam-matory disease causes a foul-smelling discharge of pus from the woman's vagina. Also, the rate of miscarriage is higher in women who have had pelvic infections.

4 *Woman cursed among her people:* Especially in biblical times was fertility the sign of a good wife and a woman blessed by God. Gonorrheal pelvic infection is one of the main causes of infertility. So the woman would not only be held in reproach for her immediate sickness, but she would suffer continuing scorn for her inability to conceive.

5 *The undefiled woman would "be free and shall conceive seed."* Unaffected by gonorrhea, the woman who had not been adulterous would not get sick and would continue to become pregnant.

The Law of Jealousy was applied only to women. The double standard functioned during biblical times as today. But the biblical recognition that the "woman shall bear her iniquity"[2] simply alleges the fact that gonorrheal infection is much more serious and easier to diagnose in women.

Venereal diseases were rampant in the ancient Mideast. Surrounding Israel were peoples whose tribal worship incorporated promiscuous sexual rites. God gave Israel strict sexual and quarantine laws which helped control the spread of such venereal diseases as syphilis, gonorrhea, *Trichomonas vaginalis,* and *Lymphogranuloma venerum* among His people.

A specific law was made, however, for the control of infectious discharges from men—discharges strongly suggestive of tuberculosis or urethral drainage from gonorrhea. The law is classic in the history of infectious disease control:

Every bed on which the man with a discharge lies down shall be ritually unclean, and everything on which he sits shall be unclean. Any man who touches the bed shall wash his clothes, bathe in water and remain unclean till evening. Whoever sits on anything on which the man with a discharge has sat shall wash his clothes, bathe in water and remain unclean till evening. Whoever touches the body of the man with a discharge shall wash his clothes, bathe in water and remain unclean till evening. If the man spits on one who is ritually clean, the latter shall wash his clothes, bathe in water and remain unclean till evening. Everything on which the man sits when riding shall be unclean. Whoever touches anything that has been under him shall be unclean till evening, and whoever handles such things shall wash his clothes, bathe in water and remain unclean till evening. Anyone whom the man with a discharge touches without having rinsed his hands in water shall wash his clothes, bathe in water and remain unclean till evening. Any earthenware bowl touched by the man shall be smashed, and every wooden bowl shall be rinsed with water.

When the man is cleansed from his discharge, he shall reckon seven days to his cleansing, wash his clothes, bathe his body in fresh water and be ritually clean.[3]

Phallic worship was prohibited by forbidding the people from falling "into the degrading practice of making figures carved in relief, in the form of a man or a woman."[4]

All idolatry was prohibited in the Ten Commandments,[5] and especially were the Israelites warned against letting their sons and daughters intermarry with the heathen and "go wantonly after their gods."[6]

The temptation of fertility worship was too great for the early Israelites. God had forseen this and had given warning of the diseases which would follow such sexual perversions. The people would be stricken "with Egyptian boils and with tumors, scabs, and itches," which would be incurable. They would have "madness, blindness, and bewilderment."[7]

Upon entering Canaan the Israelites soon "turned wantonly to worship other gods and bowed down before them."[8] Jeremiah traced the history of his people, and lamented that they had committed whoredom on "every hill-top and under every spreading tree."[9] These were the common locations for centers of fertility cult worship.

Not only had the people been warned against idolatry, but adultery[10] and prostitution[11] were proscribed on threat of death. In Proverbs, young men are warned against the seductive ways of evil women:

> I glanced out of the window of my house,
> I looked down through the lattice,

and I saw among simple youths,
there amongst the boys I noticed
a lad, a foolish lad,
passing along the street, at the corner,
stepping out in the direction of her house
at twilight, as the day faded,
at dusk as the night grew dark;
suddenly a woman came to meet him,
dressed like a prostitute, full of wiles,
flighty and inconstant,
a woman never content to stay at home,
lying in wait at every corner,
now in the street, now in the public squares.
She caught hold of him and kissed him;
brazenly she accosted him and said,
'I have had a sacrifice, an offering, to make
and I have paid my vows today;
that is why I have come out to meet you,
to watch for you and find you.
I have spread coverings on my bed
of coloured linen from Egypt.
I have sprinkled my bed with myrrh,
my clothes with aloes and cassia.
Come! Let us drown ourselves in pleasure,
let us spend a whole night of love;
for the man of the house is away,
he has gone on a long journey,
he has taken a bag of silver with him;
until the moon is full he will not be home.'
Persuasively she led him on,
she pressed him with seductive words.
Like a simple fool he followed her,
like an ox on its way to the slaughter-house,
like an antelope bounding into the noose,
like a bird hurrying into the trap;

> he did not know that he was risking his life
> until the arrow pierced his vitals.

> But now, my son, listen to me,
> attend to what I say.
> Do not let your heart entice you into her ways,
> do not stray down her paths;
> many has she pierced and laid low,
> and her victims are without number.
> Her house is the entrance to Sheol,
>   which leads down to the halls of death.[12]

The first epidemic of venereal disease to strike the Israelites likely occurred following the worship of the golden calf. The calf—a symbol of fertility—had been molded by the rebellious Israelites while Moses was on Mount Sinai receiving laws from God. Proclaiming the idolatrous object to be their deliverer from Egypt the people came to worship before the calf, "to eat and drink and then gave themselves up to revelry."[13] To restore order to the camp Moses had three thousand of the worst offenders slain. Apparently, an epidemic of venereal disease also followed when "the Lord smote the people for worshipping the bull-calf."[14]

A major outbreak of venereal disease struck the Israelites following their prostitution with the women of Moab. Joining in the worship of Baal of Peor "the people began to have intercourse with Moabite women, who invited them to the sacrifices offered to their gods."[15] So blatant was the whoredom that one of the Israelites brought a pagan woman next to the Sanctuary. The two were executed on the spot. But the plague which had struck Israel had already killed twenty-four thousand persons.[16] Moses records that those who died were the men who participated in the worship of the fertility cult,[17] thus identifying the plague as venereal. Also giving proof of this understanding by Moses is the order which he gave that all the women worshipers of Baal who had intercourse were to be killed.[18] Only these drastic measures and the imposition of a strict quarantine[19] controlled the dreadful epidemic.

Syphilis in a virulent form could account for the epidemic Israel experienced on the plain of Moab. And other descriptions given by biblical writers seem to fit the clinical pattern of this venereal disease caused by the spirocete, *Treponema pallidum.* Some of the skin diseases alluded to in Leviticus[20] may well have been the cutaneous manifestations of syphilis. As mentioned previously baldness came to the prostitutes in Isaiah's day.[21] Some have suggested that the multiple complaints of Job[22] and David[23] bespeak syphilis.

Congenital syphilis may have been alluded to by God in the Third Commandment when He proclaimed that children would be punished "for the sins of the fathers to the third and fourth generations."[24] Stigmata of congenital syphilis are well described in those persons with blindness, stunting, or bone malformations dating from birth,[25] in the macerated stillbirth "whose flesh is half eaten away when it comes from the womb,"[26] and in the children who had crooked teeth because of the sins of their fathers.[27]

Scripture References for Chapter 10

1   Numbers 5:27, 28 KJV
2   Numbers 5:31 KJV
3   Leviticus 15:4–13 NEB
4   Deuteronomy 4:16 NEB
5   Exodus 20:4, 5
6   Exodus 34:16 NEB
7   Deuteronomy 28:27, 28 NEB
8   Judges 2:17 NEB
9   Jeremiah 3:6 NEB
10 Leviticus 20:10

11 Leviticus 19:29
12 Proverbs 7:6–27 NEB
13 Exodus 32:6 NEB
14 Exodus 32:35 NEB
15 Numbers 25:1, 2 NEB
16 Numbers 25:8, 9
17 Deuteronomy 4:3, 4
18 Numbers 31:15–18
19 Numbers 31:19–24
20 Leviticus 15
21 Isaiah 3:16, 24
22 Job 7:5; 19:9; 30:17; 17:1
23 Psalms 38
24 Exodus 20:5 NEB
25 Leviticus 21:18–20
26 Numbers 12:12 NEB
27 Jeremiah 31:29

11

OBSTETRICS AND GYNECOLOGY

Childbirth, Women and Their Afflictions

And Adam said, This is now bone of my bones, and flesh of my flesh: she shall be called Woman, because she was taken out of Man.[1]

With this cryptic statement the world received its first wife, mother, lover, childbearer, and the bundle of special needs and problems upon which obstetrics and gynecology is based.

The place of women in the Bible is sometimes misunderstood by those who do not realize the low estate in which most women were held by peoples contemporary with the sacred record. In those heathen nations surrounding Israel little thought was given to preserving the life of a female infant—a point which made death by exposure a not uncommon practice for newborn females. Women living past childhood in heathen tribes could look forward to a short life-span filled with the hardships of near slavery. In contrast, the high position given men in the Bible in no way detracts from the great respect paid to the mother of the race, Eve, and to her daughters through all time.

Eve, of course, achieved fame—or infamy—early in the biblical record when she accepted the fruit offered to her by the Tempter. But notably the record did not consign her to physical servitude because of her wrong, but only to the eventuality of the pangs of childbirth. The Lord made it very specific that it would be man's responsibility to wrest his family's living from the soil: "And to the man he said, 'you shall gain your bread by the sweat of your brow until you return to the ground.' "[2]

There is no doubt but that the Bible recognizes childbearing and motherhood as the highest callings of a woman. It is of interest that in at least one text the Hebrew word for the uterus, *raham,* is translated as woman (damsel, KJV; wench, NEB) signifying the close relationship in thought between womanhood and childbearing.[3]

Infertility was looked upon as a curse and the ability to bear children as a special favor of God. Typical was the infertility of Hannah, the wife of Elkanah during the time Eli was prophet in Israel. So concerned was she over her failure to conceive that she promised God that "if thou wilt deign to take notice of my trouble and remember me, if thou wilt not forget me but grant me offspring, then I will give the child to the Lord for his whole life."

With the prophet Eli's assurance that her wish would be granted Hannah went home. "Elkanah had intercourse with his wife Hannah, and the Lord remembered her. She conceived, and in due time bore a son, whom she named Samuel."[4]

The most famous case of conception taking place after a considerable length of infertility is that of Sarah, the wife of Abraham. God had taken Abraham out beneath the clear Palestinian night sky, directed him to look at the numberless stars, and promised him that "so many shall your descendants be."[5]

But how was this to be? Surely it was not through Abraham's illegitimate son, Ishmael, born to the Egyptian woman, Hagar.

The Lord again came to Abraham with the promise of a son through Sarah. Now Abraham was one hundred years old and Sarah was ninety years of age.

Both Abraham and Sarah had grown very old, and Sarah was past the age of child-bearing. So Sarah laughed to herself and said, "I am past bearing children now that I am out of my time.'[6]

But the record is that Sarah conceived and gave birth to Isaac at the age of ninety.[7]

Of obstetrical interest is not Sarah's ninety years at a time of somewhat increased life-span over the present. But Sarah's conception was plainly postmenopausal.

There are cases recorded of conception taking place in women who are menopausal. In those cases it is apparent that periodic postmenopausal ovulation has occurred. These are extremely uncommon.

Sarah and Abraham would understandably consider the birth of Isaac to be based on God's miracle-working power.

The uterus (womb) was recognized by the ancients of biblical times as the place where babies were formed. God was given credit for the miracle of fetal formation: "Thou it was who didst fashion my inward parts; thou didst knit me together in my mother's womb."[8] God's intervention in fetal formation was not mistaken by the Jewish people as the man's role in conception. The necessity for male-female intercourse to precede pregnancy is well recognized in the Bible.

Two instances of intrauterine fetal movement are recorded in the Bible. The first is that of the twin pregnancy of Rebekah, Isaac's wife. "And the children struggled together within her."[9]

Of possibly greater significance were the intrauterine fetal movements experienced by Elizabeth, the mother of John the Baptist. Mary, already pregnant and bearing Jesus, had gone to visit her cousin Elizabeth:

And when Elizabeth heard Mary's greeting, the baby stirred in her womb. Then Elizabeth was filled with the Holy Spirit and cried aloud, 'God's blessing is on you above all women, and his blessing is on the fruit of your womb. Who am I, that the mother of my Lord should visit me? I tell you, when your greeting sounded in my ears, the baby in my womb leapt for joy.'[10]

The pangs of labor were very real to the women of biblical times without the benefit of anesthetic techniques. Scriptures describe in about thirty places either actual labor pain or allude to it allegorically as a form of severe trial and distress.

The pronouncement God made to Eve after her sin in the Garden of Eden has great obstetrical significance.

To the woman he said, 'I will increase your labour and your groaning, and in labour you shall bear children,'[11]

The Bible looks upon the fall of mankind into sin as a fall from perfectness to degeneracy. This included physical degeneracy. Significant, then, is the fact that God's pronouncement to Eve was not vindictive judgement but a statement of fact—women under the curse of sickness would develop physical problems which would hinder labor and make its pain more intense.

The normal female pelvic bones are in a configuration classified as gynecoid. This structural type, which is conducive to easy passage of the infant during labor, is determined mainly by heredity and the correct production of female hormones. It is assumed that Eve would have had a perfectly gynecoid pelvis. Her imperfect daughters to the present time would be cursed with variants of pelvic morphology which would "increase your labour and your groaning."

Also, various diseases coming with the fall of man caused increased morbidity and mortality in childbirth. These would include tuberculosis of the spine, infantile paralysis, and fractures of the pelvis.

The prophet Jeremiah evidently was an astute medical observer as judged by the number of references he made to medical situations. Interestingly he wrote six centuries before Christ one of the elemental facts of labor—first labors are more difficult than a woman's subsequent labors: "I hear a sound as of a woman in labour, the sharp cry of one bearing her first child."[12]

One could only surmise how many women Christ saw in labor or if he saw any deliveries. His description of the anguish of labor pain contrasted to the joys of the immediate postpartum period are only fully understood by those who have attended deliveries and have seen a mother's tears of pain turn to happiness with the delivery of her child. "A woman in labour," Christ observed, "is in pain because her time has come; but when the child is born she forgets the anguish in her joy that a man has been born into the world."[13]

One of the best descriptions of labor and childbirth in the Bible is found in the Book of Revelation where the birth of Christ is symbolically portrayed:

> Next appeared a great portent in heaven, a woman robed with the sun, beneath her feet the moon, and on her head a crown of twelve stars. She was pregnant, and in the anguish of her labour she cried out to be delivered. Then a second portent appeared in heaven: a great red dragon with seven heads and ten horns; on his heads were seven diadems, and with his tail he swept down a third of the stars in the sky and flung then to the earth. The dragon stood in front of the woman who was about to give birth, so that when her child was born he might devour it. She gave birth to a male child, who is destined to rule all nations with an iron rod. But her child was snatched up to God and his throne.[14]

Ezekiel probably described basic care of the newborn as he told what was not done in a neglected childbirth:

This is how you were treated at birth: when you were born, your navel-string was not tied, you were not bathed in water ready for the rubbing, you were not salted as you should have been nor wrapped in swaddling clothes. No one cared for you enough to do any of these things or, indeed, to have any pity for you; you were thrown out on the bare ground in your own filth on the day of your birth.[15]

Mention of the special newborn clothing—swaddling clothes—is further made in the Bible in the ageless description of the birth of Christ. At that fateful moment Mary took the newborn Jesus, "wrapped him in swaddling clothes, and laid him in a manger; because there was no room for them in the inn."[16]

Little is given in the Bible as to the obstetrical methods employed. It is well settled that midwives were widely used for childbirth. Several references in the Old Testament bear out this point,[17] the most interesting of which is the command of the Pharaoh of the Exodus to the Hebrew midwives to commit infanticide on all newborn Jewish males.

And the king of Egypt spake to the Hebrew midwives . . . When ye do the office of a midwife to the Hebrew women, and see them upon the stools; if it be a son, then ye shall kill him; but if it be a daughter, then she shall live.[18]

The literal meaning of "the stools" is "two stones." Egyptian birthstools consisted of either two stones or stones laid in the shape of a horseshoe. A common Egyptian saying for giving birth was: "To sit on the bricks."

The Hebrew midwives disregarded the edict of the Pharaoh and reported to him that they were not able to reach the Hebrew women in time "because the Hebrew women are not as the Egyptian women; for they are lively, and are delivered ere the midwives come in unto them."[19] Two explanations could be given for the rapid labors of the Jewish women compared to their Egyptian counterparts. First, the Israelites were evidently multiplying faster than the Egyptians. This would make a higher number of multiparous births among the Jewish women and, hence, the more rapid labor characteristic beyond the first baby. Second, some have suggested that because of unhealthful living, the Egyptian women had more disease complicating pregnancy, labor, and delivery—therefore lengthening their average time in labor.

The only mention of the placenta in the Bible is in Deuteronomy where God prophetically warned the people of the terrible conditions they would get themselves into if they ceased to follow Him. God predicted that the people would undergo such starvation that the normally delicate woman of Israel "will not share with her own husband or her son or her daughter the afterbirth which she expels, or any boy or girl that she may bear. She will herself eat them secretly in her extreme want, because of the dire straits to which you will be reduced when your enemy besieges you within your cities."[20] Not an unwarranted prophecy, it was fulfilled during three sieges: of Samaria by the Assyrians, of Jerusalem by Nebuchadnezzar, and of the dreadful onslaught against Jerusalem by Titus and the Roman legions.

Among the many public health laws given to Israel by God through Moses was an injunction against women having sexual intercourse for forty to seventy days following childbirth.[21] This undoubtably prevented many cases of postpartum endometritis or infection and injury to the healing generative organs at a time in history when antibiotics and hospitalization were not available for complications of delivery.

Major obstetrical complications were undoubtably common and took their fearful toll of maternal and infant lives. The Bible, a book written by real persons about the very real predicaments of humanity, did not fail to mention some of the problems related to pregnancy and childbirth.

Miscarriage or stillbirth is spoken of many times in the Scriptures. When Job lamented his pathetic condition he questioned:

> Why was I not still-born,
> Why did I not die when I came out of the womb?
> Why was I ever laid on my mother's knees
> or put to suck at her breasts?
> Why was I not hidden like an untimely birth,
> like an infant that has not lived to see the light?[22]

Recognizing that injury to a pregnant woman sometimes causes miscarriage, the very modernistic compensation laws given by Moses awarded damages in such cases: "When, in the course of a brawl, a man knocks against a pregnant woman so that she has a miscarriage but suffers no further hurt, then the offender must pay whatever fine the woman's husband demands after assessment."[23]

Uterine inertia complicating delivery is mentioned under two circumstances in the Old Testament. At a time of extreme national crisis during the reign of King Hezekiah the leaders of Judah acknowledged their inability to handle the situation in a message to the prophet Isaiah:

> This day is a day of trouble for us, a day of reproof and contempt. We are like a woman who has no strength to bear the child that is coming to the birth.[24]

Of even more obstetrical interest is the case of Rachel, the second wife of Jacob. Rachel was on a journey and evidently full term in her pregnancy. "And when there was still some distance to go to Ephrathah, Rachel was in labour and her pains were severe. While her pains were upon her, the midwife said, 'Do not be afraid, this is another son for you.' Then with her last breath, as she was dying, she named him Ben-oni [that is, "Son of my ill luck"] but his father called him Benjamin."[25] In this classic case description of difficult labor, delivery, and maternal mortality some very calculated speculations can be made. First, labor was apparently initiated by the work of traveling. In modern obstetrics Rachel would have been advised to not go on a long, difficult journey so close to the time of her delivery.

From the details in this description it is also observed that Benjamin was born breech. This is apparent from the fact that the midwife informed Rachel that she was bearing a son before he was completely delivered—a point which could only be correctly diagnosed by examining the genitalia of a breech infant.

In obstetrics it is well known that difficult labors such as Rachel experienced with her breech delivery are commonly followed by poor contraction of the uterus. This allows massive bleeding from the uterus. Very likely Rachel hemorrhaged fatally.

A second case of maternal mortality at the time of delivery is recorded in 1 Samuel. Here the wife of Phinehas, Eli's son, went into sudden labor when she heard that both Phinehas and Eli had died. "She crouched down and was delivered. As she lay dying, the women who attended her said, 'Do not be afraid; you have a son,' But she did not answer or heed what they said."[26] This death also appears to have been the result of prolonged bleeding following delivery.

Two instances of twin births lend depth to the study of obstetrics in the Bible. In the case of Rebecca the twins, Esau and Jacob, caused very distressful intrauterine movements. To account for this she was told by the Lord:

> Two nations in your womb,
> two peoples, going their own ways from birth!
> One shall be stronger than the other;
> the older shall be servant to the younger.[27]

This was an apt description of the lives of Jacob and Esau.

Conjectured about the birth of Jacob and Esau is the possibility that this was the first case recorded from antiquity of twin-to-twin transfusion syndrome. Of Esau it was observed that he "came out red."[28] Implied in this description was the pallor of Jacob. This condition develops occasionally from unequal vascular flow to twins through an unevenly developed monozygotic placenta.

In Genesis is also recorded the twin pregnancy and delivery of Tamar. This is also an unusual case of fetal malpresentation which was documented in a very interesting fashion by the midwife.

> When her time was come, there were twins in her womb, and while she was in labour one of them put out a hand. The midwife took a scarlet thread and fastened it round the wrist, saying, 'This one appeared first,' No sooner had he drawn back his hand, than his brother came out and the midwife said, 'What! you have broken out first!' So he was named Perez. Soon afterwards his brother was born with the scarlet thread on his wrist, and he was named Zerah.[29]

Tagging the hand of Zerah with a string probably gave him greater rights in the family system which stressed the firstborn even though Perez actually was delivered first. Perez is a Hebrew word for "breaking out." This might imply that Tamar suffered either a very rapid delivery with Perez or a perineal laceration.

Breast-feeding either by the mother[30] or by a wet nurse[31] is mentioned many times in Scripture. Wet nurses were probably employed by the wealthy or nobility, but were essential in the instances of insufficient milk formation by the mother. This was recognized as one of two serious obstetrical problems in Hosea—the other being miscarriage.[32]

Weaning was a major event in childhood during biblical

times, so much so that Isaac "was weaned, and on the day of his weaning Abraham gave a feast."[33]

Nursing had one major effect in addition to nourishing the newborn infant. It is indirectly recognized in the Bible as a form of birth control. Of the prophet Hosea's wife we have the record that "after weaning Lo-ruhamah, she conceived and bore a son."[34]

It is known today that in a number of instances the nursing mother does not ovulate and is therefore infertile. But this is definitely not a completely sure method of contraception today. However, from the viewpoint of a Creator who built into women a perfectly balanced hormonal system, nursing was probably at one point in history a perfect form of contraception. It is likely that God created the breast, pituitary, and ovarian hormonal axis in a highly sensitive balance which would prevent the conception of additional offspring until weaning had taken place and the young infant was able to be nourished away from the maternal breast.

There is no way of knowing the average family size during the various centuries of biblical history. Two Old Testament references give seven as the general number of offspring.[35] But, in the Bible the number seven is widely used in the sense of completeness or in an allegorical manner as in these two references.

Although far more space is devoted to obstetrics in the Bible than to gynecology, this latter special area is not neglected in Scripture.

As with women of all ages, biblical women menstruated with the many problems that this involves. But as today, women sometimes use the monthly menstrual flow as an excuse to dismiss themselves from unwelcome activity, so Rachel used the same ruse some four thousand years ago. Her father was searching the belongings of Jacob for several household gods which the heathen Laban used in his worship. Rachel put the gods in a camel-bag and sat on the bag. When

Laban came to her tent "Rachel said to her father, 'Do not take it amiss, sir, that I cannot rise in your presence: the common lot of woman is upon me.' "[36]

A menstruating woman was held to be ceremonially and physically contaminated according to Levitical law. Recognizing the normal menstrual flow to be somewhat less than seven days, the normal period of contamination (impurity) was listed as seven days. If, however, her menstrual flow or abnormal vaginal bleeding lasted longer than seven days, the Jewish woman was impure for as long as her bleeding continued. Sexual relations were prohibited during menstrual flow or vaginal bleeding and could not be resumed until seven days after bleeding ceased. Any object or article of clothing which was touched by menstrual flow was contaminated and had to be washed.[37]

The genius of the Mosaic law dealing with menstrual flow and other vaginal bleeding gives added support to the inspiration of the Levitical health laws. The following points relating to this law could not have been guessed by Moses or anyone else of his time without the addition of unsound aspects. It has been modern medicine's surprise to find these facts were known so long ago:

1 It is medically recognized—especially in areas of poor social hygiene—that sexual relations should be avoided during menstruation because of the greater susceptibility of the female generative organs to infections such as venereal diseases during that time.

2 To consider blood from the vagina as a contaminant requiring washing of anything it touched simply relates to the fact that blood is an excellent culture material for bacteria. It would also attract insects and other disease transmitters.

3 God had promised His people that if they followed His laws they would be more fertile than the heathen peoples in

the surrounding nations. This was partially guaranteed by prohibiting sexual relations until the fourteenth day of the menstrual cycle—basically the day the normal woman ovulates
and is most fertile.

Menorrhagia has one notable place in Scripture for a woman
suffering from this malady was miraculously cured by Christ.
Jesus was on the road traveling to heal the daughter of Jairus
who lay dying. The record is that "while Jesus was on his way
he could hardly breathe for the crowds."

> Among them was a woman who had suffered from haemor-
> rhages for twelve years; and nobody had been able to cure
> her. She came up from behind and touched the edge of his
> cloak, and at once her haemorrhage stopped. Jesus said,
> 'Who was it that touched me?' All disclaimed it, and Peter and
> his companions said, 'Master, the crowds are hemming you
> in and pressing upon you!' But Jesus said, 'Someone did touch
> me, for I felt that power had gone out from me.' Then the
> woman, seeing that she was detected, came trembling and
> fell at his feet. Before all the people she explained why she
> had touched him and how she had been instantly cured. He
> said to her, 'My daughter, your faith has cured you. Go in
> peace.'[38]

There could be many possible causes for this woman's hemorrhage. Endometrial or cervical carcinoma was probably not
the cause because of her living twelve years with the disease.
A logical diagnosis would be leiomyoma (fibroids) of the
uterus.

Whatever the cause of the woman's vaginal bleeding, it is
noteworthy that power flowing from the Master Healer accomplished for her what modern medicine would have to do
with major surgery.

Scripture References for Chapter 11

1 Genesis 2:23 KJV
2 Genesis 3:17, 19 NEB
3 Judges 5:30
4 1 Samuel 1:11, 20 NEB
5 Genesis 15:5 NEB
6 Genesis 18:12 NEB
7 Genesis 21:1–3
8 Psalms 139:13 NEB
9 Genesis 25:22 KJV
10 Luke 1:41–44 NEB
11 Genesis 3:16 NEB
12 Jeremiah 4:31 NEB
13 John 16:21 NEB
14 Revelation 12:1–5 NEB
15 Ezekiel 16:4, 5 NEB
16 Luke 2:7 KJV
17 1 Samuel 4:20
18 Exodus 1:15, 16 KJV
19 Exodus 1:19 KJV
20 Deuteronomy 28:56, 57 NEB
21 Leviticus 12:1–8
22 Job 3:11, 12, 16 NEB
23 Exodus 21:22 NEB
24 Isaiah 37:3 NEB
25 Genesis 35:16–18 NEB
26 1 Samuel 4:19, 20 NEB
27 Genesis 25:23 NEB
28 Genesis 25:25 NEB
29 Genesis 38:27–30 NEB
30 1 Samuel 1:23
31 Genesis 35:8
32 Hosea 9:14
33 Genesis 21:8 NEB

12

WINE AND WINEBIBBERS

Alcohol and Its Effects

Few nontheological subjects found within the covers of the Bible have caused more controversy than has that of alcohol. Does the Bible condemn or condone the use of alcohol? Do the Scriptures speak of moderate imbibing or medicinal intake only? In Christ's first miracle at Cana of Galilee did water become fresh grape juice or fermented wine? These and many other questions have been the basis of centuries of debate.

Alcohol, its use, and action are mentioned over two hundred times in the Bible. There is no question but that the Bible and its writers recognized the actions of alcohol on the human body—especially upon the functions of the gastrointestinal tract and the central nervous system with its motor and mental capabilities.

The nauseated drunk is not limited to modern times. Jeremiah the prophet commanded allegorically: "Make Moab drunk—he has defied the Lord—until he overflows with his vomit and even he becomes a butt for derision."[1] Isaiah described the corrupt leadership of Egypt in his day and warned that they would mislead Egypt "as a drunkard will miss his footing as he vomits."[2] Again, Isaiah gave an appropriate description of those made ill from drink in speaking of the condition of some of the priests:

> These too are addicted to wine,
>   clamouring in their cups:
> priest and prophet are addicted to strong drink
>   and bemused with wine;
> clamouring in their cups, confirmed topers,
>   hiccuping in drunken stupor;
> every table is covered with vomit,
>   filth that leaves no clean spot.[3]

Drunkenness is pictured in Scripture as a condition leading to evil acts and regrettable situations. Noah's drunken stupor with its consequences is recorded in Genesis 9:20–27. Lot became incestuously involved with his two daughters while under the influence of alcohol.[4] Belshazzar, king of the Babylonian empire after his father Nebuchadnezzar, held a drunken orgy using the Lord's temple vessels as drinking cups. On that fateful night the revelry was suddenly stopped with handwriting on the wall bearing the message:

> . . . God has numbered the days of your kingdom and brought it to an end; you have been weighed in the balance and found wanting; and your kingdom has been divided and given to the Medes and Persians.[5]

Because of these inherent abuses, alcoholic beverages were strictly denied by God to those of leadership, both religious and civil. Of the priests God commanded through Aaron:

> You and your sons with you shall not drink wine or strong drink when you are to enter the Tent of the Presence, lest you die.[6]

Lemuel penned the verity that his mother taught him:

> It is not for kings, O Lemuel, not for kings to drink wine nor for princes to crave strong drink.[7]

The Nazarites were not to becloud their minds and actions with alcohol as in the case of Samson.[8] Because of the importance of his mission as the messenger preparing the way for Christ, John the Baptist was to "never touch wine or strong drink."[9]

Paul informed Timothy that church deacons should not be given "to excessive drinking."[10] And he informed Titus that older women should not be "slaves to strong drink."[11] Daniel and his companions refused to drink alcohol in the court of Babylon's King Nebuchadnezzar.[12]

The physiologic actions of alcohol and its medical uses are correctly mentioned in the Bible. Reference has already been made of the action of alcohol on the vomiting centers of the brain. Other centers of the brain are also affected by alcohol as is so aptly pointed out in the Bible.

Before frank drunkenness comes, a person drinking alcohol passes through a state of euphoria, abandonment, and occasionally cheerfulness. This is reflected in Zechariah's declaration; "They shall be roaring drunk as with wine."[13]

As the level of alcohol in the bloodstream increases, levity gives way to a loss of motor control—a fact the Bible mentions many times. "They reeled and staggered like drunken men."[14]

Even as motor control is lost, alcohol anesthetizes the brain so that the memory centers are affected:

Give strong drink to the desperate and wine to the embittered; such men will drink and forget their poverty and remember their trouble no longer.[15]

Alcohol intake can lead to the point of death either from overintoxication or illnesses which can attack the body when resistance is low. This fact biblical writers recognized: "Drink this, get drunk and be sick; fall, to rise no more."[16] "I will cause their drinking bouts to end in fever and make them so drunk that they will writhe and toss, then sink into unending sleep, never to wake."[17]

Not only are the physiologic effects of alcohol on the body correctly described in the Bible, but medicinal uses for alcohol were mentioned and recommended. As medicine alcohol seems to have been correctly prescribed in the Bible.

The alcoholic content of wine probably made it the best antiseptic known to the ancients. In prescribing wine for wound-cleansing, biblical people were using an antiseptic which is still the most common ingredient of modern surgical skin-scrubbing solutions. In giving the classic medical parable of the Good Samaritan, Christ told that when the Samaritan came upon the dying man "he went up and bandaged his wounds, bathing them with oil and wine."[18]

Alcohol is not best given for all stomach conditions. But it is a well-known stimulant of the appetite. Although Paul never claimed to be a knowledgeable medical diagnostician, he probably was giving Timothy the best medical advice of his day when he wrote: "Stop drinking nothing but water; take a little wine for your digestion, for your frequent ailments."[19] Luke the physician was a frequent companion of Paul. It is interesting to speculate that Paul's advice to Timothy might have actually been suggested by Luke.

Medically the tranquilizing effects of alcohol are well known and were apparently widely used by biblical peoples. Solomon counseled that those who were deeply distressed should be given "strong drink" so that they would "remember their trouble no longer."[20]

Those who stood at the Crucifixion during Christ's last suffering followed the custom of offering Him wine. At first Christ turned down the benumbing mixture[21] but as death approached He said: " 'I thirst.' A jar stood there full of sour wine; so they soaked a sponge with the wine, fixed it on a javelin, and held it up to his lips. Having received the wine, he said, 'It is accomplished!' He bowed his head and gave up his spirit."[22]

Two other instances of Christ coming into contact with wine

have been widely debated. The first instance was His turning water into wine at a wedding feast in Cana of Galilee. All that is stated of this miracle is that the wine Christ made was of superior quality to that which had been previously provided for the guests.[23]

While preaching on one occasion Christ referred to the alcoholic action of "new wine" which would produce carbon dioxide while fermenting and cause internal pressure to build in the wine container.

> Neither do you put new wine into old wine-skins; if you do, the skins burst, and then the wine runs out and the skins are spoilt.[24]

In instituting the Lord's Supper, Christ passed wine to His disciples as a symbol of the blood sacrifice He was about to offer.

> Then he took a cup, and after giving thanks he said, 'Take this and share it among yourselves, for I tell you, from this moment I shall drink from the fruit of the vine no more until the time when the kingdom of God comes.'[25]

Highly fermented wine would seem to have been out of context with the Passover service which Christ was celebrating because of the impurity associated with fermentation. However, there is no question that some members of the early Christian Church used fermented wine in their celebration of the Lord's Supper. Paul had to soundly condemn the drunkenness associated with celebration of the Lord's Supper at the Corinthian church. He pointed out that the Corinthians' gluttony and drunkenness was "why many are feeble and sick, and a number have died."[26]

There is no question that both Old and New Testament writers condemned drunkenness and the inherent evils of alcohol. Paul warned the Ephesians to "not give way to drunkenness and the dissipation that goes with it."[27] Solomon observed that "wine is an insolent fellow, and strong drink makes an uproar; no one addicted to their company grows wise."[28]

And, it was the wisdom of Solomon which gave to the world one of the greatest descriptions of the effects of alcoholic addiction:

> Whose is the misery? whose the remorse?
> Whose are the quarrels and the anxiety?
> Who gets the bruises without knowing why?
> Whose eyes are bloodshot?
> Those who linger late over their wine,
> those who are always trying some new spiced liquor.
> Do not gulp down the wine, the strong red wine,
> when the droplets form on the side of the cup;
> in the end it will bite like a snake
> and sting like a cobra.
> Then your eyes see strange sights,
> your wits and your speech are confused;
> you become like a man tossing out at sea,
> like one who clings to the top of the rigging;
> you say, 'If it lays me flat, what do I care:
> As soon as I wake up,
> I shall turn to it again.'[29]

Scripture References for Chapter 12

1   Jeremiah 48:26 NEB
2   Isaiah 19:14 NEB
3   Isaiah 28:7, 8 NEB
4   Genesis 19:30–38
5   Daniel 5:26–28 NEB
6   Leviticus 10:8, 9 NEB

7   Proverbs 31:4 NEB
8   Judges 13; Numbers 6:1–4
9   Luke 1:15 NEB
10 1 Timothy 3:8 NEB
11 Titus 2:3 NEB
12 Daniel 1:8–16
13 Zechariah 9:15 NEB
14 Psalms 107:27 NEB; *see also* Job 12:25;
    Isaiah 19:14
15 Proverbs 31:6, 7 NEB
16 Jeremiah 25:27 NEB
17 Jeremiah 51:39 NEB
18 Luke 10:34 NEB
19 1 Timothy 5:23 NEB
20 Proverbs 31:6, 7 NEB
21 Matthew 27:34
22 John 19:28–30 NEB
23 John 2:2–11
24 Matthew 9:17 NEB
25 Luke 22:17, 18 NEB
26 1 Corinthians 11:17–30 NEB
27 Ephesians 5:18 NEB
28 Proverbs 20:1 NEB
29 Proverbs 23:29–35 NEB

13

WHATSOEVER YOU EAT OR DRINK

Diet

Better a dish of vegetables if love go with it than a fat ox eaten in hatred.[1]

The Bible becomes to the interested a looking glass wherein is reflected history, legend, literature, and religious ritual. But from the pages of the Bible are also illuminated surprisingly specific details of everyday life as they concerned the peoples of antiquity. Hygiene, sex, birth, death, and even daily eating habits became the expressions of biblical writers.

Biblical teaching closely correlates good diet with both health and the religious life. "Well," concluded the Apostle Paul, "whether you eat or drink, or whatever you are doing, do all for the honour of God."[2]

Daniel had centuries before brought this principle into practical application as he begged his Babylonian captors to give him and his Hebrew companions food approved in the Mosaic health code. "Submit us to this test for ten days. Give us only vegetables to eat and water to drink; then compare our looks with those of the young men who have lived on the food assigned by the king, and be guided in your treatment of us by what you see."[3] Abstaining from unclean foods and wine the four Hebrew worthies prospered during the ten days, and "they looked healthier and were better nourished than all the young men who had lived on the food assigned them by the king."[4] This was Daniel's first victory in a political career which saw him become a privileged counselor for two world kingdoms.

Daniel's training was based on the rather specific Mosaic dietary code. But biblical concern with man's eating habits goes beyond Moses to the table set before Adam and Eve in the Garden of Eden. To them God said, "I give you all plants that bear seed everywhere on earth, and every tree bearing fruit which yields seed: they shall be yours for food."[5]

Meat is not found in the biblical record as part of the Edenic diet. Though some might view the diet given to Adam and Eve as having been rather stringent, it apparently was conceived to give man direct nutrients. As such early man would receive proteins, carbohydrates, and bulk from nuts and grains, minerals and vitamins from fruits and greens, and vegetable fats from a variety of sources.

Although man's habits undoubtably changed before then, no record of God having changed dietary laws is found until Noah descended from the Ark to the flood-ravaged earth. With plant life in an array of destruction God told Noah: "Every creature that lives and moves shall be food for you; I give you them all, as once I gave you all green plants."[6]

But it was not without price that man turned to animals for food after the Flood.

"The fear and dread of you shall fall upon all wild animals on earth, on all birds of heaven, on everything that moves upon the ground and all fish in the sea."[7]

Man hunted animals for food. Man himself would fall prey to wildlife—both to their savagery and to their diseases. The intermingling of animal diseases more intimately with mankind might have helped bring about the dramatic decrease in life-span which was noted to have occurred shortly after the Flood.

One command by God after the Flood was reiterated in the health laws given to the Israelites of the Egyptian Exodus. Although meat was for human consumption, blood was not to be eaten.[8] Though this had significance in the biblical respect for blood as a symbol of life, it also helped prevent the spread of blood-borne animal diseases to man.

Another restriction of the Levitical health laws prohibited the eating of animal fat although the fat could be used for domestic needs such as lamp fuel.[9] A strict command, its violation by the sons of Eli was a reason for God's mortal judgment against them.[10]

Viewed from the perspective of modern medicine the prohibition against eating animal fat had great epidemiological significance. By adhering to this law God's people would have a lower incidence of arteriosclerosis and thereby a lower death rate from such conditions as heart attack and stroke. Arteriosclerosis plagued ancient man as it does his modern counterpart, as is evidenced by the finding of typical fatty deposits in the arteries of Egyptian mummies.

The most profound of the Levitical laws governing the eating of meat was that which differentiated between the unclean and clean animals. The unclean animals were not to be eaten. This law covered the eating of mammals, sea life, and birds. Medically the law was a sound control in the spread of infectious diseases as it divided nonhuman life into two groups: scavengers and nonscavengers. Not to be eaten—or even touched—were the scavengers which found their own sustenance in eating dead animals and the wastes of other creatures. Insects and reptiles were, in general, included among the prohibited scavengers.[11] Placing the law in tabular form makes its applications clear.

THE MOSAIC SEPARATION OF CLEAN AND UNCLEAN FOODS BASED ON LEVITICUS 11 AND DEUTERONOMY 14

CRITERIA	CLEAN	UNCLEAN
ANIMALS		
Clean animals must chew the cud and have cloven hooves. Animals which had only one or neither of these features ere unclean. Clawed animals were unclean.	cattle deer goats sheep	pigs badgers, wolves, mink camels bears, cats, lions
WATER CREATURES		
Clean sea life must have both scales and fins. Creatures with scales but not fins or creatures with fins but not scales were unclean.	perch trout bass salmon	shellfish sharks catfish
BIRDS		
Clearly scavenger birds were made unclean.	chickens pigeons doves	vultures falcons owls crows bats (a mammal)
OTHERS		
Most insects and reptiles were unclean.		

Of all the unclean animals none was more abhorred than the pig. Specifically stated to be unclean for food or handling in the Levitical laws[12] swine are particularly disdained throughout the Bible. "Those who eat the flesh of pigs and rats and all vile vermin, shall meet their end, one and all, says the Lord," Isaiah prophesied.[13]

Christ cast devils into a herd of swine causing them to run into the Sea of Galilee and drown.[14] On another occasion Christ depicted the depraved condition of the prodigal son who came to the bottom of his riotous living by tending pigs.[15] And Solomon wrote his Proverb of the pig:

> Like a gold ring in a pig's snout is a beautiful woman without good sense.[16]

In prohibiting the Israelites from eating swine, God protected them from contacting the many diseases directly transmitted to man from pigs. Common among these diseases are trichinosis caused by the parasite, *Trichinella spiralis,* and the pig tapeworm, *Taenia solium.* With pigs prohibited from among the people, infectious vectors such as contaminated water and insects would also be less.

Also assuring a higher degree of health among the Israelites was the prohibition against eating or touching anything which had died from an illness or from attack by another animal.[17] This law, with its inherent inspiration and medical genius, greatly reduced the spread of infectious diseases among God's people.

In addition to these laws, the Bible records special diets or meals such as the Passover,[18] the manna in the wilderness,[19] the diet of John the Baptist,[20] and Christ's Last Supper.[21]

Scripture References for Chapter 13

1   Proverbs 15:17 NEB
2   1 Corinthians 10:31 NEB
3   Daniel 1:12, 13 NEB

4   Daniel 1:15 NEB
5   Genesis 1:29 NEB
6   Genesis 9:3 NEB
7   Genesis 9:2 NEB
8   Genesis 9:4; Leviticus 7:26
9   Leviticus 7:22–25
10   1 Samuel 2:12–17
11   Leviticus 11:1–30; Deuteronomy 14:3–20
12   Leviticus 11:7
13   Isaiah 66:17 NEB
14   Matthew 8:28–32
15   Luke 15:11–16
16   Proverbs 11:22 NEB
17   Leviticus 11:8, 24, 28, 32–40
18   Exodus 12
19   Exodus 16
20   Matthew 3:4; Luke 1:15
21   Matthew 26:26–29

14

A VIRGIN SHALL CONCEIVE

The Medical Enigma of Jesus Christ

This is the story of the birth of the Messiah. Mary his mother was betrothed to Joseph; before their marriage she found that she was with child by the Holy Spirit. Being a man of principle, and at the same time wanting to save her from exposure, Joseph desired to have the marriage contract set aside quietly. He had resolved on this, when an angel of the Lord appeared to him in a dream. "Joseph, son of David," said the angel, "do not be afraid to take Mary home with you as your wife. It is by the Holy Spirit that she has conceived this child. She will bear a son; and you shall give him the name Jesus (Saviour), for he will save his people from their sins." All this happened in order to fulfill what the Lord declared through the prophet: "The virgin will conceive and bear a son, and he shall be called "Emmanuel", a name which means "God is with us." Rising from sleep Joseph did as the angel had directed him; he took Mary home to be his wife, but had no intercourse with her until her son was born.[1]

In those days a decree was issued by the Emperor Augustus for a registration to be made throughout the Roman world. This was the first registration of its kind; it took place when Quirinius was governor of Syria. For this purpose everyone made his way to his own town; and so Joseph went up to Judaea from the town of Nazareth in Galilee, to register at the city of David, called Bethlehem, because he was of the house of David by descent; and with him went Mary who was betrothed to him. She was expecting a child, and she gave birth to a son, her first-born. She wrapped him in his swaddling clothes, and laid him in a manger, because there was no room for them to lodge in the house.[2]

To become embroiled in the argument over the nature of the birth of Christ seems futile, indeed. Already nineteen centuries old, that debate is as enduring as the biblical story is ageless. It is true that Isaiah 7:14 in the King James Version, "Behold, a virgin shall conceive, and ear a son," is translated in modern versions such as in the New English Bible, "A young woman is with child, and she will bear a son." But New Testament writers interpreted the prophecy as referring to a virginal woman, and attributed such a miraculous situation to the birth of Christ.

Of course it is well recognized that fertilization can take place without actual male penetration of coitus. The biblical record, however, does not imply this as the cause of Mary's pregnancy. The conception of Christ is plainly stated to have been a miracle involving Mary and Deity.

Christ's actual birth has fascinated all Christians. Artists have attempted to capture the setting. Poets have given it an aura. And historians have contributed chronologies, geographical details, and the social setting of that age.

The medical story of Christ's birth appears to have been uncomplicated. It is likely that the trip from Nazareth to Bethlehem was difficult for Mary as she was near the time of delivery. Its rigors might have even contributed to the start of her labor. Because of the lack of other facilities Christ was born in an animal shelter. But such a location might not have been any worse than the birthplaces of other first-century infants of the same economic status. Mary was prepared for Christ's birth for she had the necessary swaddling clothes in which He was placed.

An obvious miracle associated with the birth of Christ was that he survived the delivery and newborn period—especially in an animal shelter. The low survival rate of infants in ancient times is well documented even when their births took place under optimal conditions. A particular scourge for newborns in unsanitary locations was (and continues to be) tetanus. Commonly called "lockjaw," tetanus is a rapidly fatal disease of the nerves caused by a toxin from the organism, *Clostridium tetani*. This organism is most often found in the feces of such animals as cows, sheep, and horses. It was, therefore, likely present in large numbers in the animal shelter and even the manger occupied by the newborn Jesus.

A healthy newborn, Christ was circumcised and named Jesus at eight days of age.[3] Then, following forty days of Mary's healing as ordered in Levitical law, Jesus was taken to the temple in Jerusalem to be dedicated to God.[4]

The first months of Christ's life were spent in Egypt where his family had fled to avoid the persecution of Herod, king of Judea. After Herod died, Joseph, Mary, and Jesus returned to Nazareth.[5] Here Christ as a child "grew big and strong and full of wisdom."[6] Despite the lack of formal education Christ astounded the temple teachers with His knowledge during a Passover visit to Jerusalem when He was twelve years old.[7]

Christ was "about thirty years old"[8] when He was baptized in the Jordan River by John the Baptist. This was also the start of Christ's three-and-one-half years of public ministry.

Following His baptism, Christ went into a wilderness area for forty days of fasting. Although assuring the devil during this time that "man cannot live on bread alone"[9] Christ ended the ordeal "famished."[10] Weakened, "angels appeared and waited on him."[11]

As a real Person, the historical Christ shared the physiology of mankind. He was physically healthy and strong as a result of years of carpentry work. His ministry was that of a wanderer —adding to His physical fitness as He walked the trails of the Holy Land. Christ's strength was demonstrated on two occasions when He frightened raucous merchants into fleeing from the temple.[12]

Despite physical strength Christ became exhausted in His work. Once while crossing the Sea of Galilee during a storm so severe that His disciples feared for their lives, Christ fell asleep.[13] On another occasion He sought a quiet place where He and the disciples could rest.[14]

Christ appreciated good food and was often invited to eat in the homes of friends, the inquisitive, or opportunists. His social habits brought the accusation that He was "a glutton and a drinker."[15] He recognized the nutritional needs of others as especially evidenced when He miraculously provided bread and fish for a multitude of hungry persons.[16]

Christ demonstrated the spectrum of human emotions. He had compassion for the sick.[17] The essence of His teaching was love, a principle He practiced and instilled in His followers. "I give you a new commandment: love one another; as I have loved you."[18] Christ knew grief. When his friend Lazarus died, "Jesus wept."[19]

It was a mere three-and-one-half years of public work which made Christ the single greatest force in the parade of human history. Volumes have been written to attempt to explain the phenomenon of Jesus the Christ.

His work as a teacher gives some insight into Christ's greatness. The parables which He spoke gave ageless lessons as in the Parable of the Good Samaritan where every man discovers the identity of his neighbor.[20]

Christ became profoundly eloquent when He spoke of what is and what should be. Nothing attests to this more than His matchless Sermon on the Mount. Of this sermon the record rightly states: "When Jesus had finished this discourse the people were astounded at his teaching."[21]

Through His public ministry Christ became loved by children, the sick, and those whose lives He changed. He was understood by the ignorant, and respected by the intelligent. Christ knew the situation of all He met. He lovingly lifted children to His lap. Nicodemus received one of Christ's great sermons in the solitude of the night. The psychology of sin proved no mystery to Christ as He meted out new lives to the woman taken in adultery and the woman at the well. And the workings of the human mind came into full review when Christ scathingly rebuked the hypocritical.

The claim of divine power in the work of Christ is nowhere more evident than in His work as a healer. Invoking the power of God, Christ made the paralyzed walk, restored sight to the blind and hearing to the deaf, and revitalized the flesh of lepers. And in the ultimate display, the dead received life from the Master Healer.

As His work progressed, Christ's path led inexorably towards death on the cross. Hated by the religious leaders, proclaimed by the people as the deliverer from Roman rule, and feared by the Romans as a potential king, Christ made His final entry to Jerusalem on the Sunday of Crucifixion Week amid the noisy adulations of the Passover crowds. The early part of the Passion Week was spent by Christ in the last few acts of public ministry—including His last visit to the temple.

Thursday night Christ celebrated the Passover with the twelve disciples. Here He instituted the Lord's Supper by washing the disciples' feet and offering wine and bread as the symbols of His soon-to-be-spilled blood and broken body.

After Judas left the supper on his errand of betrayal, Jesus and the eleven retired to the seclusion of Gethsemane, a garden on the slope of the Mount of Olives. Here, while the disciples slept, Christ prayed to God for strength for the coming conflict. With such anguish did He pray that "his sweat was like clots of blood falling to the ground."[22] (Hematidrosis, the excretion of blood or blood products in the sweat, is a rare medical phenomenon.)

Suddenly the night's quietness was pierced by sounds of the crowd sent to capture Christ. Led to Christ by the betrayal kiss of Judas, the captors were about to accomplish their purpose when Peter swung out with his sword. He severed the right ear of Malchus, a servant of the High Priest. This incongruous setting was the scene of Christ's last miraculous healing. Turning to Malchus, Christ "touched the man's ear and healed him."[23]

During that night's incarceration Christ was repeatedly beaten[24] as was also the case during the trials of the next day.[25] At one time Christ was left to the wiles of the Roman soldiers guarding Him.

> They stripped him and dressed him in a scarlet mantle; and plaiting a crown of thorns they placed it on his head, with a cane in his right hand. Falling on their knees before him they jeered at him: 'Hail, King of the Jews!' They spat on him, and used the cane to beat him about the head.[26]

It was in violation of Roman law that Pilate allowed the flogging of Christ—still declared innocent of any crime by the Roman prelate. That was not the only usurpation of justice which occurred during the three trials of Christ. The accusation of the Sanhedrin that Christ had committed blasphemy was disallowed by Pilate, a recognition of acquittal. Twice Pilate declared Christ's innocence of the charge of treason. And both Pilate and Herod acquitted Christ of sedition.

After futile attempts to placate the raucous clamor of the crowd Pilate finally released a convicted criminal, Barabbas, from prison and handed Christ over for crucifixion. Knowing of Christ's innocence of any crime worthy of death Pilate "took water and washed his hands in full view of the people, saying, 'My hands are clean of this man's blood; see to that

yourselves.' "[27] So in the crossing of two of the most enlight-
ened systems of law the world had ever known Jesus the Christ
began the long journey to the cross without having been convicted of a crime.

The air over Jerusalem was heavy on that Preparation Friday. It was not merely the day before the Sabbath; it was the
Preparation for the Passover Sabbath. The Passover crowds
became absorbed in the drama as this Galilean preacher—
burdened by the weight of His own cross—was led toward the
spot of execution, a hill called Golgotha. Christ, having gone
without sleep or food, was also weakened by floggings and
loss of blood. Seeing Christ's condition, the Roman guards
interned a foreigner, Simon, to bear the cross.

At noon on that Friday Christ was crucified.

An execution practiced by the ancients on the worst crimi-
nals, crucifixion was feared as a cruel form of death. The
finding of a crucifixion victim amid excavations in Jerusalem
has clarified the actual mechanics of this mode of capital punishment. Still clearly visible on this two-thousand-year-old
skeleton are the marks of spikes which had been driven between the radial and ulnar bones of the forearm and through
the calcaneal bones of the heels. To prevent the victim's
weight from tearing him from the impalement the cross included a seat for support.

At first refusing to drink a drug offered to stupify the pain,[28]
Christ asked for it as His death approached.[29] Slipping into
deeper shock from pain and loss of blood, "Jesus again gave
a loud cry, and breathed his last."[30]

To verify that Christ was dead a Roman soldier "stabbed his
side with a lance, and at once there was a flow of blood and
water."[31]

Christ's burial was accomplished before sundown marked
the beginning of the Sabbath. Two friends of Christ, Joseph of
Arimathea and Nicodemus buried Him in a new garden tomb.
Using "a mixture of myrrh and aloes . . . they took the body

of Jesus and wrapped it, with the spices, in strips of linen cloth according to Jewish burial-customs."[32]

Jesus lay dead in the tomb over the Sabbath. The biblical account of His Resurrection is concise. The women who viewed the open tomb on that Resurrection morning were told:

> He is not here; he has been raised again, as he said he would be."[33]

Jesus was seen by many for over a month after the Resurrection. They viewed the marks of His Crucifixion,[34] ate with Him,[35] and received His last messages of encouragement and instruction.[36]

His ministry finished, Christ took the disciples to the Mount of Olives where, "as they watched, he was lifted up, and a cloud removed him from their sight."[37]

Scripture References for Chapter 14

1   Matthew 1:18–25 NEB
2   Luke 2:1–7 NEB
3   Luke 2:21
4   Luke 2:22
5   Matthew 2:19–23
6   Luke 2:40 NEB
7   Luke 2:41–52
8   Luke 3:23 NEB
9   Luke 4:4 NEB
10 Luke 4:2 NEB
11 Matthew 4:11 NEB
12 John 2:13–16; Matthew 21:12–16
13 Matthew 8:23–27
14 Mark 6:30, 31

15 Matthew 11:19 NEB
16 Mark 6:30–44
17 Matthew 9:36
18 John 13:34 NEB
19 John 11:35
20 Luke 10:30–37
21 Matthew 5–7; Matthew 7:28 NEB
22 Luke 22:44 NEB
23 Luke 22:51 NEB
24 Luke 22:63–65
25 Matthew 27:26
26 Matthew 27:28–30 NEB
27 Matthew 27:24, 25 NEB
28 Matthew 27:33, 34
29 John 19:28, 29
30 Matthew 27:50 NEB
31 John 19:34 NEB
32 John 19:39, 40 NEB
33 Matthew 28:6 NEB
34 John 20:26–29
35 John 21:1–13
36 John 21:15–22
Matthew 28:18–20
Acts 1:1–8
37 Acts 1:9 NEB

15

THE MASTER HEALER

The Miracles of Christ

Miracles have intrigued man since time began. This has been manifest by man's fascination with such productions of nature as lightning, thunder, the movements of the sun, moon, and stars, and the forces in wind, water, or fire.

But in the condition of man possibly nothing has elicited such amazement and respect as the victory of healing against apparently incurable diseases.

Of course, the miraculous is always relevant to the time of its occurrence. As the ancients deified the unknown forces of nature, modern man has studied and at times controlled those same forces. And in the battle against sickness, that which appeared miraculous even a few generations ago is now accepted with concerted casualness.

But in the miraculous healings of Christ are found not only the triumph of the unknown to the people of His day, but aspects which transcend the finite to make modern man stand in respect. For the recorded miracles of Christ give an element of completeness which even medicine today does not enjoy: perfect sight was restored, the lame became runners, lepers found wholeness, and the insane conquered full reality.

And to Christ was attributed the ultimate in power over the human predicament: He raised the dead to life.

The miracles of Christ will always cause wonderment and discussion. It would seem that the only plausible way to approach such a subject would be to accept the witnesses to Christ's miracles as honest recorders of what they saw. What they recorded can then be evaluated in the light of modern medicine.

The competence of the recorders of Christ's miracles need not have been inept. For evidence is strong that one such chronicler was a physician schooled in the rather observant character of Greek medicine. Luke, the physician, wrote of the miracles of Christ in such a manner as to add credulity to both the recorded history and the acts of the Master Healer.

Although twenty-six medically related miracles are described and attributed to Christ, it is to be noted that His work as a physician consumed a major part of His three-and-one-half-year ministry. Without giving details, the New Testament several times claims that Christ healed the sick throughout whole communities.[1] It is without wonder, then, that the Apostle John would write of Christ:

> And there are also many other things which Jesus did, the which, if they should be written every one, I suppose that even the world itself could not contain the books that should be written.[2]

Christ recognized the necessary function of the physician. "It is not the healthy that need a doctor," Christ said one day, "but the sick."[3] But in the healings of Christ we find the working of One unlike the common physician of the first century. As the Master Healer, Jesus Christ and the miracles He performed dominate medicine in the New Testament.

> And sufferers from every kind of illness, racked with pain, possessed by devils, epileptic, or paralyzed, were all brought to him, and he cured them.[4]

Possibly no diseases have so distressed mankind as those impinging upon the functions of the brain and the nervous system. Neurological disease, regardless of its manifestation, has been an object of both awe and frustration from man's first recognition of it to the present. Until the advent of modern medicine, illness of the nervous system has often been attributed to demon possession. This was so in New Testament times.

Mental illness has often been misunderstood and its sufferers mistreated. One such man "possessed by an unclean spirit" dwelt among the tombs of Gadara. Psychotic with mania, "he could no longer be controlled; even chains were useless; he had often been fettered and chained up, but he had snapped his chains and broken the fetters. No one was strong enough to master him. And so, unceasingly, night and day, he would cry aloud among the tombs and on the hill-sides and cut himself with stones."[5] Christ healed the maniac and left him "clothed and in his right mind."[6]

Frightening in its manifestations is grand mal epilepsy. The violent seizures of those so afflicted often cause injury from falls or a bitten tongue. Suffocation is not uncommon. Following a grand mal seizure the victim lapses into a comalike state from which he usually arises. Christ healed a boy who had been epileptic from "childhood." His epilepsy could have been caused by birth injury, a childhood head injury, or an infection in the brain. The symptoms, as described by the boy's father to Jesus, are classic of epilepsy. The attack, stated the distraught father, "makes him speechless. It dashes him to the ground, and he foams at the mouth, grinds his teeth, and goes rigid. Often it has tried to make an end of him by throwing him into the fire or into water."[7]

Other cures by Christ of persons suffering neurological disease attributed to "demon" possession were: the demoniac in the synagogue,[8] the dumb demoniac,[9] the blind and dumb demoniac,[10] and the Syrophoenician woman's daughter.[11]

Paralysis is often devastating because without the ability to walk or use other body parts a person becomes dependent on others for care and material support. For this reason the crippled persons Christ saw were particularly pathetic in their illnesses and joyous in their healings.

Amid the colonnades bordering Jerusalem's pool of Bethesda many sick persons gathered with the hope that the supposed magic of its waters would some day heal them. "Among them was a man who had been crippled for thirty-eight years."[12] Jesus met the cripple and heard of the duration of his malady. The age of the cripple is not given. Possibly an accident during his youth severed his spinal cord, or polio might have struck him down. Regardless, it was Christ's command, "Rise to your feet, take up your bed and walk,"[13] which erased the suffering of thirty-eight years.

Many of Christ's healings were done on the Sabbath to show that the Sabbath was designed for the benefit of man. On one Sabbath Christ healed a woman who had been crippled for eighteen years. She suffered from a deformity of the spine, kyphosis, for "she was bent double and quite unable to stand up straight."[14] Her deformity could have been caused by such conditions as a broken back, aging, or tuberculosis.

Another Sabbath healing was of a man with a "withered arm."[15] Nothing more than this apt description of paralysis and muscle wasting is needed to diagnosis this man's illness as polio.

An acute case of spinal meningitis is apparent in the son of a Roman centurion who was "paralyzed and racked with pain."[16] Christ healed the boy in a demonstration of the faith of this foreign soldier.

A paraplegic restored to health by Christ was the Capernaum man who was lowered on his bed through a roof to where Christ was talking to a crowd.[17]

Although spread of leprosy was controlled among the Jews because of the strict Levitical health laws, it remained an endemic curse among them as with other peoples of the ancient Mediterranean world. The health laws given by God through Moses provided a crude method for diagnosing early leprosy even though other skin diseases might mimic it. For this reason the priests were given the position of health-wardens and allowed to expel from the communities persons known to have this dread disease. The priests could also judge if a leper had been cursed.[18]

Disfigured by his spreading disease, the leper became an outcast beggar—avoided by all.

The New Testament records that Christ healed lepers on two occasions. Eleven men were thereby cured. Having cured one leper, Christ asked him to take the required purification offering and go to the priests to "certify the cure."[19]

Ten lepers approached Christ another time. "They stood some way off and called out to him, 'Jesus, Master, take pity on us.' When he saw them he said, 'Go and show yourselves to the priests'; and while they were on their way, they were made clean."[20]

Christ declared; "The spirit of the Lord is upon me because he has anointed me; he has sent me to announce good news to the poor, to proclaim release for prisoners and recovery of sight for the blind; to let the broken victims go free."[21]

In extending the compassion of His healing touch, no miraculous act could have pleased the Saviour more than restoring sight to the blind. Blindness in Christ's day was extremely common—yet devastating in its consequences. Not only were the blind reduced to rank poverty, but their beggarly state was abhorred by others. Blindness was considered evidence of God's disfavor. This was not the case, assured Christ when He healed a man who had been blind since birth.

The Sabbath healing of this man was done so that "God's power might be displayed in curing him."[22]

In this case of healing it is possible that the blind man had been rendered sightless during the first few weeks of life because of *ophthalmia neonatorum. Ophthalmia neonatorum* — or gonorrheal conjunctivitis—was very common during biblical times. In this disease the eyes of the infant are infected with the bacteria, *Neisseria gonorrhoeae,* while passing through the mother's birth canal.

When Christ healed the blind a miracle took place. But on two occasions He placed a mud paste on the sightless eyes before cure was accomplished.[23] That this was an accepted treatment for eye conditions during New Testament times is illustrated in the condition of the church at Laodicea which was spiritually "blind." The church was advised to buy "ointment" for its eyes and be cured.[24]

> In truth, in very truth I tell you, a time is coming, indeed it is already here, when the dead shall hear the voice of the Son of God, and all who hear shall come to life.[25]

To conquer death has been a dream of medicine since the most ancient mystic droned incantations over the dead. In the medical ministry of Christ claim is made for three instances where He brought back to life those who had crossed the chasm of death.

The New Testament records that the twelve-year-old daughter of Jairus arose from her bed of death at Christ's command.[26] In a similar fashion Christ stopped a funeral procession bearing the deceased son of a widow of Nain, and resurrected the dead man from the bier.[27]

But it is in the story of the resurrection of Lazarus by Christ that medical drama in the New Testament achieves its highest point. Lazarus, a brother of Mary and Martha, was a beloved friend of Jesus. Jesus was laboring near Perea when He heard of Lazarus's mortal illness. This was some twenty miles from the home of Lazarus in Bethany. By the time Christ arrived in Bethany Lazarus had died, been ceremonially prepared, and "had already been four days in the tomb."[28]

With Bethany only two miles from Jerusalem, Christ recognized this chance of not only assuaging the grief of Mary and Martha but also demonstrating to the people the divine nature of His mission.

"Your brother will rise again," Christ assured Martha.

Arriving at the tomb of Lazarus Christ ordered that its stone door be removed. Aware of the rapid decomposition of bodies in the heat of Judea, Martha protested. "Sir, by now there will be a stench."[29] Insisting that the stone be removed, Christ stepped before the open tomb.

> Then he raised his voice in a great cry: 'Lazarus, come forth.' The dead man came out, his hands and feet swathed in linen bands, his face wrapped in a cloth.[30]

Scripture References for Chapter 15

1   Luke 6:17–19; 7:21–23
2   John 21:25 KJV
3   Matthew 9:12 NEB
4   Matthew 4:24 NEB
5   Mark 5:2–6 NEB
6   Mark 5:15 NEB
7   Mark 9:17, 18, 22 NEB
8   Mark 1:21–28
9   Matthew 9:32–34
10 Matthew 12:22–32
11 Matthew 15:21–28
12 John 5:5 NEB
13 John 5:8 NEB
14 Luke 13:11 NEB
15 Mark 3:1–5
16 Matthew 8:6 NEB
17 Mark 2:1–12

18　Leviticus 13; 14
19　Matthew 8:4 NEB
20　Luke 17:12–14 NEB
21　Luke 4:18 NEB
22　John 9:3 NEB
23　Mark 8:23
　　 John 9:6, 7
24　Revelation 3:14–22
25　John 5:25 NEB
26　Mark 5:22–24, 35–43
27　Luke 7:11–16
28　John 11:17 NEB
29　John 11:39 NEB
30　John 11:43, 44 NEB

16

THE GOOD SAMARITAN

Who Is My Neighbor?

The parables of Christ alone are enough to assure Him a place of greatness for all time. With these stories He led the people through simple words to great themes. Among Christ's parables stands one so telling in its simplicity and power that its message speaks to all men of all time. It is the Parable of the Good Samaritan. This parable also must be placed at the point where the healing arts find their most satisfying moments.

The Parable of the Good Samaritan arose from a question directed at Christ by a Jewish lawyer. "Master, what must I do to inherit eternal life?" When it was pointed out that the sum of the law was to "love the Lord your God with all your heart, with all your soul, with all your strength, and with all your mind; and your neighbour as yourself," the lawyer posed the ageless question: "Who is my neighbour?"[1]

It was no erudite definition which Christ gave the lawyer— simply a story. And the story became a definition of "my neighbor" which has lived for two thousand years. As Jesus told the story:

'A man was on his way from Jerusalem down to Jericho when he fell in with robbers, who stripped him, beat him, and went off leaving him half dead. It so happened that a priest was going down by the same road; but when he saw him, he went past on the other side. So too a Levite came to the place, and when he saw him went past on the other side. But a Samaritan who was making the journey came upon him, and when he saw him was moved to pity. He went up and bandaged his wounds, bathing them with oil and wine. Then he lifted him on to his own beast, brought him to an inn, and looked after him there. Next day he produced two silver pieces and gave them to the innkeeper, and said, "Look after him; and if you spend any more, I will repay you on my way back." Which of these three do you think was neighbour to the man who fell into the hands of the robbers?' He answered 'The one who showed him kindness.'[2]

Most of the details of the story Christ told were well known by the lawyer and the rest of the audience. The road between Jerusalem and Jericho went through desolate country where lone travelers were often attacked, beaten, and robbed.

The characters making up the story have always been important because of the attitudes prevalent in Christ's day and still with us today. The "half-dead" victim of the robbery was an unknown traveler beaten and bruised beyond recognition. The priest and the Levite were both bound under Mosaic law to be the health officers of Israel. Theirs was not only a humanitarian privilege to stop and help the dying stranger, but also a divinely given responsibility. The Samaritan, on the other hand, was from a nationality despised by the Jews because of centuries of religious animosities. He would appear to have been the last person willing to stop and help someone who was most likely a dying Jew.

The reasons for the priest and Levite not stopping to give needed care were not given by Christ. They might have feared attack by the same robbers. Perhaps they were on a hurried errand of great importance. Possibly they did not wish to become contaminated—either physically or ceremonially. Only they knew the score of excuses as they hurried past the point of potential involvement with a fellow human being. But their excuses really do not matter in the story which Christ told, for his story was not about them but about the Good Samaritan.

No details were given by Christ about the Samaritan's station in life or urgency in traveling. Of the Samaritan it was only made clear that when he saw the dying man he was "moved to pity."

Few descriptions of actual medical treatment are found in the Bible. But when Christ told of the Good Samaritan, physician Luke recorded the details of correct medical care.

The Good Samaritan cleansed the wounds with wine—giving needed antisepsis through the antibacterial action of the alcohol. Then soothing oil was placed on the wounds and they were tenderly bandaged.

With no ambulance service running between Jerusalem and Jericho the Good Samaritan transported the dying man on the best available conveyance—his "beast." Taking the victim to the nearest inn the Good Samaritan paid for the stranger's further care.

The greatness of the Parable of the Good Samaritan is the fact that in reality it is the story of Everyman. No person who has ever walked the face of the earth has not been in the position of the one robbed, wounded, and forsaken. As such Everyman had known sickness, heartache, mental illness, financial destitution, loss of relatives from death or physical separation, or any of the hundreds of distresses uniting us all into the human predicament.

But Everyman was not only the "neighbor" left to die on the road between Jerusalem and Jericho. In the parable—and in life—all act the part of passing by those in need of our ministrations. And to Everyman come those moments of decision whether he will pass on by without offering help, or whether he will answer the call coming from the Master Teacher to be the Good Samaritan.

Scripture References for Chapter 16

1   Luke 10:25–29 NEB
2   Luke 10:30–37 NEB

17

LUKE, THE BELOVED PHYSICIAN

Journalist and Historian

Into the early Christian Church entered a man who was to have profound effect upon that group, the recording of its history, and the saga of New Testament medicine. His name was *Loukas* in the Greek language of the first century Mediterranean world. Today he is recalled as Luke.

Little is known of Luke's background. Early Christian tradition holds him to have been a citizen of Antioch in Syria. Internal evidence of the New Testament suggests that Luke was a non-Jewish convert to the Christian Church.[1] He apparently was soon engulfed in the activities of the Church; especially through the close friendship which formed between him and the great Apostle Paul.

Luke became the foremost historian of the early Christian Church. Only Paul contributed more of the writings which became the New Testament. Early Church writers and tradition unanimously attribute to Luke the authorship of the Gospel which bears his name. Luke's Gospel was the first of a two-volume history of the Church, the second volume being the Book of Acts.[2] The Gospel of Luke deals with the life of Christ while Acts chronicles events in the expanding work of that Church founded by Christ.

Not a personal witness to the ministry of Christ, Luke traveled over Palestine interviewing those who had seen Christ work or had been healed by Him. Biblical scholars acknowledge Luke to have been a careful historian—the detail of his record bears this out.

The evidence for Luke having been a physician is compelling. Medicine of the first-century Mediterranean world was dominated by Greek thought. Greek medicine of that time is known for its meticulous descriptions of disease. Luke's tutelage in Greek medicine lend status to the veracity of his observations on medical situations in the New Testament. It is possible that Luke attended the famous medical school at Tarsus near Antioch.

Evidence within the Book of Acts and in Paul's writings indicate that Luke spent lengthy periods of time with Paul. Luke first joined Paul at Troas during the apostle's second missionary journey.[3] Paul had just come from Galatia where he had founded Christian churches. While at Galatia Paul seems to have had a worsening of the illness which afflicted his eyes[4] —a situation which might have prompted Luke the physician to come to Troas to treat Paul. Luke traveled with Paul to Philippi[5] where Luke stayed, and where they again met near the end of Paul's third missionary trip.[6]

Luke accompanied Paul to Jerusalem. Following Paul's trials in Jerusalem and Caesarea, Luke again joined him for the long trip to Rome and eventual martyrdom. In letters written from his imprisonment in Rome, Paul sent greetings from himself and others including Luke.[7] It was in one such letter that Paul identified Luke as "the beloved physician."[8]

As Paul's death neared he wrote to Timothy appealing for him to come to Rome. Deserted by past friends and temporarily separated from others, Paul reminded Timothy that "I have no one with me but Luke."[9] This message stands as a fitting tribute to the loyalty of Luke to Paul—both as a friend and as a physician.

As Luke chronicled the history of his age he wrote with a skill which identifies him as having been highly educated. The Gospel of Luke was written in a style unsurpassed in the New Testament. Not only does Luke's style of writing prove his education, but the words he used plainly point out his medical training.

Luke, as a physician, used specific terms in describing illness or anatomical parts. In doing this he was more exact than the other Gospel writers. A typical example is Luke's record of Christ healing the man suffering from dropsy.[10] This is a specific medical term not used by other Gospel writers.

While other Gospel writers simply noted the withered hand, Luke wrote in good clinical detail that it was the right hand which Christ healed one Sabbath in the synagogue.[11] And while John also confirmed that Peter cut off Malchus' right ear[12] (Matthew and Mark didn't specify which ear) in the Garden of Gethsemane, Luke was the only one to record that Christ "touched the man's ear and healed him."[13]

Luke showed more awareness of physicians' limitations when he clarified Mark's description of the plight of the bleeding woman, who "in spite of long treatment by many doctors, on which she had spent all she had,"[14] had not improved. Luke merely asserted that "nobody had been able to cure her."[15]

Alone among the Gospel writers was Luke in recording the proverb which Christ spoke: "Physician, heal yourself."[16]

Two parables of Christ which dealt with medical situations were recorded only by Luke. One of these—the Parable of the Good Samaritan—stands as a classic description of good medical care and a compelling story of the compassion shown by a healer to his patient.[17] The other parable is about the rich man and Lazarus.[18] In this story of human predicament Christ dramatized the conditions of a rich man and a beggar, Lazarus, who lay at the rich man's gate. Starving, Lazarus was unable to protect himself from the dogs which licked his sores. The rich man offered to Lazarus neither food nor medical treatment. As St. Cyril observed of Lazarus: "The only attention, and, so to speak, medical dressing, which his sores received was from the dogs who came and licked them."

As would be expected from a physician, Luke recorded more of Christ's miracles of healing than did Matthew, Mark, or John.

Luke's close attention to fact and his particular position as a physician greatly enhance the reliability of the accounts of the healing miracles of Christ.

Scripture References for Chapter 17

1 Colossians 4:10–14
2 A comparison of Luke 1:1–4 and Acts 1:1, 2 confirms the common authorship of these books.
3 In Luke's account of Paul's journey the personal pronoun, "they" (Acts 16:8, 9) becomes "we" (Acts 16:10) at Troas.
4 Galatians 4:12–16; 6:11
5 Acts 16:12
6 Acts 20:6
7 Philemon 24
8 Colossians 4:14 KJV
9 2 Timothy 4:11
10 Luke 14:1–4
11 Luke 6:6
12 John 18:10
13 Luke 22:51 NEB
14 Mark 5:26 NEB
15 Luke 8:43 NEB
16 Luke 4:23 NEB
17 Luke 10:30–37
18 Luke 16:19–31

18

NEW TESTAMENT MEDICINE

An Overview

As in the Old Testament, trauma was not an unusual specter for the people living during the time of Christ and His apostles. John the Baptist's life ended by decapitation by order of Herod Antipas the Roman ruler of Galilee. John had criticized Herod for the adulterous marriage to Herodias, the wife of his half brother, Philip. Incensed at John the Baptist's intrusion in her life, Herodias had her daughter make a birthday request of Herod: "Give me here on a dish the head of John the Baptist."[1]

John the Baptist was not the only believer in Christ who sealed his ministry in death. Stephen was stoned outside of Jerusalem and became the first martyr of the infant Christian Church. Having enraged a crowd with a testimony of the Deity of Christ, Stephen went to his death crying out, "Lord, do not hold this sin against them."[2]

Witnessing Stephen's death and giving approval was a young Jew of Roman citizenship, Saul of Tarsus. Saul became a violent persecutor of Christians until his blinding conversion to that faith on the road to Damascus. With that conversion Saul's name was changed to Paul. Christianity then gained its greatest missionary.

The scene of Stephen's martyrdom must have later haunted

Paul during a mob attack in Lystra, a city of Roman Galatia. Having been incited to riot because of Paul's healings and preaching, a crowd "stoned Paul, and dragged him out of the city, thinking him dead."[3] Paul survived, however, and left the next day for the city of Derbe.

On at least one occasion Paul's preaching contributed to a serious head injury. Eutychus was a young man of Troas who attended Paul's Saturday night farewell sermon. As young men sometimes do, "Eutychus, who was sitting on the window-ledge, grew more and more sleepy as Paul went on talking. At last he was completely overcome by sleep, fell from the third story to the ground, and was picked up for dead."[4] But Eutychus was only unconscious from a brain concussion. The record is that he lived.

The medical scene of the first century A.D. contained many problems related to mental illness. An unusual condition, psychophonasthenia, afflicted Zechariah when he refused to believe that his wife would bear a son. Zechariah remained unable to speak throughout Elizabeth's pregnancy, her delivery, and until the child was named on the day of his circumcision.[5] This fascinating drama surrounded the birth of John the Baptist.

Sudden emotional shock might be implicated in the deaths of Ananias and his wife, Sapphira. Reneging on their promise to give the money from a sale of land to the church, Ananias and Sapphira dropped dead when confronted with their deceit.[6] The actual cause of their deaths was probably either heart attack or stroke. Whatever the cause, the death of this couple had a profound effect on the members of the small Christian Church.

Severely psychotic was the man in Ephesus who attacked a crowd of Paul's listeners, "overpowered them all, and handled them with such violence that they ran out of the house stripped and battered."[7] His actions fit those of a person suffering from a manic psychosis.

Classic in its relentless progress was the mental illness of Judas, one of the twelve disciples of Christ. All of the hopes, fears, and delusions which drove Judas to his fateful betrayal of Christ are not known.[8] But with that betrayal for thirty pieces of silver blood money the mind of Judas became haunted with guilt over what he had done. Frustrated in his attempts to rebuy Christ's life Judas threw down the money in the temple, "and went and hanged himself."[9] Scripture records that after the hanging Judas "fell forward on the ground, and burst open, so that his entrails poured out."[10]

With the gift of the Holy Spirit at Pentecost the followers of Christ gained the power of miraculous healings. Peter and John healed a beggar who had been born lame—possibly from either a congenital defect or brain damage caused by an inept delivery.[11] Another man crippled from birth was healed by Paul in Lystra.[12] And Philip healed "many paralysed and crippled folk" in Samaria.[13]

One man's orthopedic problem was not healed. That was Zacchaeus, the dwarf who had to climb a sycamore tree in order to see over the crowd surrounding Jesus.[14]

Infectious and parasitic diseases were a nemesis of ancient peoples. This was true in New Testament times. Christ healed Simon Peter's mother-in-law from a severe fever which was likely caused by malaria.[15] She lived in Capernaum on the edge of the Sea of Galilee—a likely spot for the breeding of mosquitos which carry malaria.

After being shipwrecked on the coast of Malta, Paul healed a man on the island who "was in bed suffering from recurrent bouts of fever and dysentery,"[16] a common scourge of the Mediterranean world.

King Herod (Agrippa I) became an archpersecutor of the early Christian Church. He ordered the death of the Apostle James by decapitation. And he imprisoned Peter.[17] But King Herod had his own health problems which became acute during a public speech at his capital, Caesarea. Mortally struck down, "he was eaten up with worms."[18] Intestinal worms have been implicated.

As with the miracles of Christ, nothing in the healings of His apostles transcended raising the dead to life. New Testament medicine is unsurpassed in the story of Tabitha:

> In Joppa there was a disciple named Tabitha (in Greek, Dorcas, meaning a gazelle), who filled her days with acts of kindness and charity. At that time she fell ill and died; and they washed her body and laid it in a room upstairs. As Lydda was near Joppa, the disciples, who had heard that Peter was there, sent two men to him with the urgent request, 'Please come over to us without delay.' Peter thereupon went off with them. When he arrived they took him upstairs to the room, where all the widows came and stood round him in tears, showing him the shirts and coats that Dorcas used to make while she was with them. Peter sent them all outside, and knelt down and prayed. Then, turning towards the body, he said, 'Get up, Tabitha.' She opened her eyes, saw Peter, and sat up. He gave her his hand and helped her to her feet."[19]

Teachings of the New Testament make it clear that Christians are to ask for and expect to receive miraculous healings in the name and power of Christ. Christ had promised His followers that "anything you ask in my name I will do. . . ."[20]

This charismatic power was but an extension of both Old Testament miracles and those of Christ. But contrasting with Old Testament reliance on the priest-healer, New Testament healing was to be brought about through the believer's faith in Christ.

Even though each true believer had within his grasp the miracle of faith healing, it was recognized in the early Christian Church that the special gifts of the Holy Spirit blessed certain individuals most specifically with the power of healing.[21]

And as Christ's representative in the world, the church organization was to be utilized in seeking the miraculous healing of the sick. Instructions were given as to how church leaders were—and are—to go about requesting divine healing of the sick: "Is one of you ill? He should send for the elders of the congregation to pray over him and anoint him with oil in the name of the Lord. The prayer offered in faith will save the sick man, the Lord will raise him from his bed, and any sins he may have committed will be forgiven. Therefore confess your sins to one another, and pray for one another, and then you will be healed."[22]

Scripture References for Chapter 18

1   Matthew 14:8 NEB
2   Acts 7:60 NEB
3   Acts 14:19 NEB
4   Acts 20:9, 10 NEB
5   Luke 1:19–22, 57–79
6   Acts 5:1–10
7   Acts 19:16 NEB
8   Matthew 26:14–25, 47–50
9   Matthew 27:5 NEB
10 Acts 1:18 NEB
11 Acts 3:1–10
12 Acts 14:8–10
13 Acts 8:8 NEB
14 Luke 19:1–4
15 Mark 1:21, 29–31
16 Acts 28:8 NEB
17 Acts 12:1–3
18 Acts 12:23 NEB
19 Acts 9:36–41 NEB
20 John 14:13 NEB
21 1 Corinthians 12:9
22 James 5:14–16 NEB

19

A THORN IN THE FLESH

Eye Diseases—Paul's and Others

Blindness was a great scourge of antiquity. Nothing attests to this fact more than the Bible.

Such a recognized part of life was blindness during Moses' time that laws were written to protect the blind: "Cursed be he that maketh the blind to wander out of the way."[1] And the code in Leviticus prohibited persons from putting "an obstruction in the way of the blind."[2]

On the other hand, the priesthood, as a representation to the people of the perfect nature of God, excluded from its membership those with physical deformity, including blindness.[3]

Lacking understanding to correct such conditions as glaucoma and senile cataract, old age was for many a period of partial or total blindness. It is possible that glaucoma was present in four elderly blind men of the Old Testament: Isaac,[4] Israel,[5] Eli,[6] and Ahijah.[7] Typical of these four was Eli who was awaiting news about the safety of his sons who were fighting against the Philistines. At the age of ninety-eight Eli "sat staring with sightless eyes." When told that his two sons had been killed and that the Ark of God had been captured in battle Eli fell backwards from his seat, suffered a broken neck, and died.[8]

Glaucoma in old age comes from a deterioration of the parts

of the eye which exchange and circulate eye fluids. Pressure builds up within the eye and causes destruction of the sensitive cells which pick up transmitted light. Just as today, senile cataract was no doubt a curse to the aged of biblical times. In this condition the lens of the eye becomes cloudy with progressive dimming of vision leading to total blindness. If Isaac suffered from cataracts he could now be cured by their surgical removal. However, this was not available to him. Using the blindness against him, Rebecca and Jacob tricked Isaac into bestowing the previous paternal blessing on Jacob instead of Esau. This started the greatest family fight of the Bible.[9]

Trachoma is an inflammatory condition of the eyes leading to blindness. It is an infectious disease caused by a virus and is especially prevalent in the biblical countries among persons with poor sanitary conditions. Leah, the "dull-eyed" first wife of Jacob might have had trachoma. The conjunctivitis of trachoma would have made her much less attractive than her sister Rachel. But as he had fooled his blind father, so was Jacob tricked into marrying Leah—the girl he did not love.[10]

A remarkable incident of increased visual acuity followed by an equally remarkable epidemic of blindness is found in 2 Kings, chapter 6. Here the Syrian (some sources: Aramaean) hosts were seiging Dothan, a city where Elisha was staying. In fear, Elisha's servant surveyed the army surrounding the city. Elisha assured his servant that "those who are on our side are more than those on theirs." Elisha then prayed that God would allow the young servant's eyes to be opened. "And the Lord opened the young man's eyes, and he saw the hills covered with horses and chariots of fire all round Elisha."

God's prophet, Elisha, then prayed again. This time the entire Syrian army was struck with blindness. The army was then led to Samaria, the capital of Israel where their sight was restored and they were fed by the astonished king. Even more astonished were the Syrian soldiers when Elisha directed that they be allowed to return unharmed to their own country.[11]

Neither of these two alterations of the sight process could be considered natural.

The most intriguing case of blindness in the Bible found its beginning the day when Stephen fell to his knees under the onslaught of stones thrown by a furious crowd. As this killing took place in Jerusalem giving the Christian Church its first martyr, the mob "laid their coats at the feet of a young man named Saul. And Saul was among those who approved of his murder."[12]

Saul was a Jewish citizen of Tarsus, an important Roman metropolis in Cilicia. He was both a Roman citizen and a member of the Jewish sect, the Pharisees.

With the martyrdom of Stephen the newly formed Christian Church entered a period of both rapid growth and violent persecution. Saul of Tarsus became chief of the persecutors— that is, until that fateful day on the road to Damascus.

The story of Saul's blinding conversion is graphic:

> While he was still on the road and nearing Damascus, suddenly a light flashed from the sky all around him. He fell to the ground and heard a voice saying, 'Saul, Saul, why do you persecute me?' 'Tell me, Lord,' he said, 'who you are.' The voice answered, 'I am Jesus, whom you are persecuting. But get up and go into the city, and you will be told what you have to do.' . . . Saul got up from the ground, but when he opened his eyes he could not see; so they led him by the hand and brought him into Damascus. He was blind for three days, and took no food or drink.[13]

The record is that after the three days of blindness a Christian named Ananias was sent to Saul where a miraculous healing took place; ". . . it seemed that scales fell from his eyes, and he regained his sight."[14]

But, did Paul (as Saul is referred to after Acts 13:9) regain all of his sight, or did he have relapses of eye disease for the rest of his life? These are questions which have challenged theologians and medical experts for centuries. And the basis for this intrigue is as interesting as it is challenging.

Paul set the stage for such a question when he indicated that God—in order to keep him from self-glorification—had given him "a bitter physical affliction . . . a very messenger of Satan, to harass me, to keep me from being too much elated" ("thorn in the flesh" in the King James Version).

This physical ailment bothered Paul enough that "three times"[15] he prayed to the Lord pleading for its removal.

Although Paul was able to travel to the far reaches of the civilized globe and undergo untold hardships for the Christ he came to love, it seems that either by choice or need he usually had medical help nearby. This was in the person of Luke, "the beloved physician,"[16] who was a close traveling companion of Paul. When Paul came to the last days of his life in Rome he could say, "I have fought a good fight, I have finished my course, I have kept the faith." His former friends had deserted him. "Only Luke," Paul said of his physician friend, "is with me."[17]

Lending credence to the possibility that partial blindness was Paul's "thorn in the flesh," is the observation that he apparently used a scribe to write most of his letters. It was not unusual for Paul to sign the letters or add a note at the end of a letter in his own handwriting. For example, Tertius penned the Epistle to the Romans for Paul.[18] And, the first letter to the Corinthians ends with a message from Paul and the assurance that "this greeting is in my own hand—Paul."[19]

But it is near the end of Galatians where the evidence accumulates as Paul again signed the letter with his own handwriting. This time, however, he acknowledged difficulty seeing what he was writing when he said, "You see these big letters? I am now writing to you in my own hand."[20]

It was also in this letter that Paul recounted his early ministry to the church in Galatia at a time when he was bothered with physical illness. That illness, he hinted, affected his eyes so much that the Galatians wished they could have given him nondiseased eyes:

> As you know, it was bodily illness that originally led to my bringing you the Gospel, and you resisted any temptation to show scorn or disgust at the state of my poor body; you welcomed me as if I were an angel of God, as you might have welcomed Christ Jesus himself. Have you forgotten how happy you thought yourselves in having me with you? I can say this for you: you would have torn out your very eyes, and given them to me, had that been possible!"[21]

The final evidence linking Paul's "thorn in the flesh" to eye disease comes from an episode which occurred during one of the several trials against him as he slowly wended his way towards Rome and martyrdom. Paul was well acquainted with the Jewish religious hierarchy in Jerusalem. He was brought before those religious leaders for trial:

> Paul fixed his eyes on the Council and said, 'My brothers, I have lived all my life, and still live today, with a perfectly clear conscience before God.' At this the High Priest Ananias ordered his attendants to strike him on the mouth. Paul retorted, 'God will strike you, you whitewashed wall! You sit there to judge me in accordance with the Law; and then in defiance of the Law you order me to be struck!' The attendants said, 'Would you insult God's High Priest?' 'My brothers,' said Paul, 'I had no idea that he was High Priest; Scripture, I know, says: You must not abuse the ruler of your people.'[22]

Not only did Paul know what Ananias looked like, but Ananias certainly was wearing the robes and jewelry which marked him as the High Priest. Yet Paul, standing in front of him, was not able to see Ananias or his clothing.

If Paul were, indeed, partially blind, we do not have sufficient evidence on which to diagnose the type of blindness. Did the blinding conversion experience near Damascus render upon Paul a permanent, partial blindness?

Medically, one condition fits the clinical history of exposure to brilliant light followed by blindness from which recovery is never complete. That is a burned retina in which the vital *macula densa* is destroyed when the eye's lens concentrates light waves coming from a bright source. This is the type of blindness sustained when an eclipse of the sun is viewed without adequate protection of the eyes.

Paul's handicap was probably a lifelong reminder of that fateful day on the road to Damascus when he encountered his Christ. But it was part of the conversion by which the Christian Church became a world force. Indeed, Paul turned handicap into victory. For Paul came to the end of his life service with the thrilling claim:

> I have fought a good fight, I have finished my course, I have kept the faith: Henceforth there is laid up for me a crown of righteousness, which the Lord, the righteous judge, shall give me at that day: and not to me only, but unto all them also that love his appearing.[23]

Scripture References for Chapter 19

1   Deuteronomy 27:18 KJV
2   Leviticus 19:14 NEB
3   Leviticus 21:18
4   Genesis 27:1
5   Genesis 48:10
6   1 Samuel 3:2, 4:15
7   1 Kings 14:4
8   1 Samuel 4:15–18 NEB

9   Genesis 27
10 Genesis 29:15–30 NEB
11 2 Kings 6:15–23 NEB
12 Acts 7:58, 60 NEB
13 Acts 9:3–9 NEB
14 Acts 9:18 NEB
15 2 Corinthians 12:7–9 NEB
16 Colossians 4:14 KJV
17 2 Timothy 4:7, 11
18 Romans 16:22
19 1 Corinthians 16:21 NEB; *see also* Colossians 4:18,
    2 Thessalonians 3:17, 18
20 Galatians 6:11 NEB
21 Galatians 4:13–16 NEB
22 Acts 23:1–5 NEB
23 2 Timothy 4:7, 8 KJV

20

HONOR THE HOARY HEAD

Aging and the Aged

The days of our years are three-score years and ten; and if by
reason of strength they be fourscore years, yet is their strength
labour and sorrow.[1]

It must have been with some frustration that the psalmist
acknowledged "three-score years and ten" as the common
end point of man's life. As David wrote those words he no
doubt recalled the books of Moses and the long life attributed
to such men as Adam (930 years), Jared (962 years), Me-
thuselah (969 years), and Noah (950 years).

The Bible records the life-span of pre-Flood man and then
the rapid decay which brought old age to less than a century.
But even with the ravages of sickness and degeneracy shorten-
ing man's life-span, Scripture presents old age as a period of
respect and productivity.

Such an implicit part of Scripture is honor for the mature that
it was written as one of the Ten Commandments: "Honour
your father and your mother, that you may live long in the land
which the Lord your God is giving you."[2] Though this text
speaks of filial responsibilities, it has been recognized as also
engendering respect for the advanced years of parents. It is of
note that this is the one commandment of the Ten to which

141

a promise was attached—a promise of eventual old age for those who obeyed.

Not just parents were to be honored, but the Torah prescribed respect for all old people. "You shall rise in the presence of grey hairs, give honour to the aged."[3] Because of this persons who became elderly were accorded places of honor and were sought out for counsel by biblical people.

However, the aging process which inexorably led to man's common enemy, death, was understandably feared by the ancients. David lived zestfully but recognized the signs of aging. His concern for the unknown end of life was expressed in a plea to God: ". . . now that I am old and my hairs are grey, forsake me not, O God."[4]

David had seen strong and good men age and face death. His friend, Barzillai, spoke forcefully to David of the personal ravages of senility:

> Your servant is far too old to go up with your majesty to Jerusalem. I am already eighty; and I cannot tell good from bad. I cannot taste what I eat or drink; I cannot hear the voices of men and women singing. Why should I be a burden any longer on your majesty? . . . Let me go back and end my days in my own city near the grave of my father and mother. . . .[5]

Unexcelled in the world's literature is Solomon's description of old age. Apparently disillusioned with the shortness of life and the frustrations of its decline Solomon counseled youth of their most certain future:

> Remember your Creator in the days of your youth, before the time of trouble comes and the years draw near when you will say, 'I see no purpose in them.' Remember him before the sun and the light of day give place to darkness, before the moon and the stars grow dim, and the clouds return with the rain

—when the guardians of the house tremble, and the strong men stoop, when the women grinding the meal cease work because they are few, and those who look through the windows look no longer, when the street-doors are shut, when the noise of the mill is low, when the chirping of the sparrow grows faint and the song-birds fall silent; when men are afraid of a steep place and the street is full of terrors, when the blossom whitens on the almond-tree and the locust's paunch is swollen and caperbuds have no more zest. For man goes to his everlasting home, and the mourners go about the streets. Remember him before the silver cord is snapped and the golden bowl is broken, before the pitcher is shattered at the spring and the wheel broken at the well, before the dust returns to the earth as it began and the breath returns to God who gave it.[6]

The symptoms of aging as chronicled by Solomon can be better appreciated when extracted:

V.	1	I see no purpose in them	Mental slowing of senility
V.	2	Sun and light of day give place to darkness, the moon and stars grow dim	Failing sight
V.	4	Look through windows no longer	Blindness
V.	3	Guardians of the house tremble	Shaking arms
V.	3	Strong men stoop	Bowing of the back and legs
V.	3	Women grinding meal cease	Death of marriage partners (or loss of teeth)
V.	4	Noise of the mill is low, the chirping of the sparrow grows faint, and the song-birds fall silent	Deafness

V.	5	Men afraid of a steep place	Loss of balance
V.	5	Street full of terrors	General fearfulness
V.	5	Blossom whitens on the almond-tree	White hair
V.	5	Locust's paunch is swollen	Enlarging of abdomen
V.	5	Caperbuds have no more zest	Loss of sexual drive
V.	6	Silver cord is snapped	Weak backbone
V.	6	Golden bowl broken	Mental illness
V.	6	Pitcher shattered at the spring and wheel broken at the well	Loss of urine and bowel control

"Emptiness, emptiness, says the Speaker, all is empty."[7]

Scripture References for Chapter 20

1 Psalms 90:10
2 Exodus 20:12 NEB
3 Leviticus 19:32 NEB
4 Psalms 71:18 NEB
5 2 Samuel 19:34, 35, 37 NEB
6 Ecclesiastes 12:1–7 NEB
7 Ecclesiastes 12:8 NEB

21

A TIME TO DIE

The Certainty of Death and the Promised Renewal

The Lord is my shepherd; I shall not want.
He maketh me to lie down in green pastures:
   he leadeth me beside the still waters.
He restoreth my soul:
   he leadeth me in the paths of righteousness for his name's
   sake.
Yea, though I walk through the valley of the shadow of death,
I will fear no evil:
for thou art with me; thy rod and thy staff they comfort me.
Thou preparest a table before me in the presence of mine
   enemies:
thou anointest my head with oil;
   my cup runneth over.
Surely goodness and mercy shall follow me all the days of my
   life:
and I will dwell in the house of the Lord for ever.[1]

For everything its season, and for every activity under heaven
its time:
   a time to be born and a time to die.[2]

To man throughout all ages nothing has seemed more certain than death. Of this inevitable specter biblical writers often

took note. "What man," asked David, "shall live and not see death?"[3]

The Bible dates the beginning of man's alliance with death back to the sin of Adam and Eve in the Garden of Eden. "Dust you are, to dust you shall return," God said to Adam following his sin of disobedience.[4]

The Apostle Paul also spoke of man's inherited appointment with death in his letter to the church in Rome.

> It was through one man that sin entered the world, and through sin death, and thus death pervaded the whole human race.[5]

Having observed murders, wars, and death directly related to immorality and intemperate living, ancient man could easily say that "sin pays a wage, and the wage is death."[6]

Death is presented in the Bible as a natural reversal of the creation of life. Even as God first breathed into man "the breath of life,"[7] so when He "takes away their breath, they fail and they return to the dust."[8] Christ, on one occasion, called death a "sleep."[9]

In the Old Testament death is viewed as a state from which man could not return despite occasional miraculous resurrections such as the Shunammite's son.[10] The Israelites were prohibited from attempting to speak to the dead[11] because death was a state without intelligence or activity. Job spoke of the dead man whose "sons rise to honor, and he sees nothing of it; they sink into obscurity, and he knows it not."[12] Solomon agreed:

> True, the living know that they will die; but the dead know nothing. There are no more rewards for them; they are utterly forgotten. For them love, hate, ambition, all are now over.[13]

Old Testament prophets looked forward to eventual triumph over death. Isaiah envisioned a time when "the Lord will swallow up that veil that shrouds all the peoples, the pall thrown over all the nations; he will swallow up death for ever."[14]

The people of the New Testament witnessed Christ raise the dead and His victory over the grave. Even as they recalled Christ's Resurrection so they were reminded of His promised return[15] and eternal life for those who believed on Him.[16] "I am the resurrection and I am life," Christ taught. "If a man has faith in me, even though he die, he shall come to life."[17]

To the New Testament Christian was brought the hope of life after death through the Resurrection. "The time is coming when all who are in the grave shall hear his voice and come out," Christ foretold.[18]

This victorious theme was echoed by the Apostle Paul:

> For the Lord himself shall descend from heaven with a shout, with the voice of the archangel, and with the trump of God: and the dead in Christ shall rise first.[19]

John the Revelator envisioned "a new earth" where "there shall be an end to death, and to mourning and crying and pain."[20]

The story of medicine in the Bible is in reality the story of Everyman. For all mankind comes into the world assured of the ravages of sickness, injury, and finally death. Medicine and the Bible have recognized man's predicaments, attempted to explain them, and hoped for eventual victory over them. Medicine's vision is in reality the vision of John the Revelator who saw a river, and "on either side of the river stood a tree of life, which yields twelve crops of fruit, one for each month of the year; the leaves of the trees serve for the healing of the nations. Every accursed thing shall disappear."[21]

Scripture References for Chapter 21

1   Psalms 23
2   Ecclesiastes 3:1, 2 NEB

3 Psalms 89:48 NEB
4 Genesis 3:19 NEB
5 Romans 5:12 NEB
6 Romans 6:23 NEB
7 Genesis 2:7 NEB
8 Psalms 104:29 NEB
9 John 11:11
10 2 Kings 4:32
11 Deuteronomy 18:9–12
12 Job 14:21 NEB
13 Ecclesiastes 9:5, 6 NEB
14 Isaiah 25:7, 8 NEB
15 John 14:1–3; Acts 1:11
16 John 3:16, 17
17 John 11:25 NEB
18 John 5:28 NEB
19 1 Thessalonians 4:16 KJV
20 Revelation 21:1, 4 NEB
21 Revelation 22:2, 3 NEB

GLOSSARY

Adultery   Sexual intercourse between a married person and someone other than the spouse.

Anesthesia   Alleviation of pain by administration of agents that block passage of pain impulses to the brain.

Arteriosclerosis   Thickening and hardening of arterial walls usually accompanied by deposits of fats.

Balanitis   Inflammation of the penis.

Bestiality   Sexual intercourse between a human and an animal.

Birthstool   A special seat commonly used throughout history by women when giving birth.

Breech   In childbirth, refers to the buttocks of the infant being expelled before the head.

Bubonic plague   A serious infectious disease caused by the microorganism, *Pasteurella pestis.*

Cancer   A malignant growth of tissue capable of local or distant extension in the body and of causing death.

Carcinoma   *See* CANCER

Castration   Surgical removal of the testicles.

Cataract   Opacification of the lens of the eye.

Cervix   The opening of the uterus into the vagina.

Cholera   A severe infectious disease caused by the microorganism, *Vibrio cholerae,* and manifest by diarrhea, vomiting, and dehydration.

Circumcision   Surgical removal of the male foreskin.

Coitus   The union of male and female in sexual relations.

Conjunctivitis   Inflammation of the mucous membrane lining of the eyelids and eye.

Consanguineous marriage   A marriage between persons of close blood relationship.

Dropsy   A large collection of fluid within the body, usually within the abdomen.

Ecology   A study of the interactions of organisms and the world's environment.

Endometrium   The mucous membrane which lines the uterus.

Epidemic   Any disease process which affects a large number of persons in an area over a short period of time.

Epilepsy   A disorder of the nervous system which in its severest form (grand mal) causes convulsions, unconsciousness, and sometimes death.

Eunuch   A male who has been castrated.

Faith healing   The miraculous healing of the sick through the power of Christ when requested by the true believer.

Gangrene   Death of tissue caused by lack of blood flow.

Glaucoma   A disease marked by increased pressure within the eye leading to the destruction of delicate cells necessary for vision.

Gonorrhea   An acute venereal infection of the genitalia caused by the microorganism, *Neisseria gonorrhoeae*.

Gout   A painful arthritis caused by the accumulation of uric acid in joints.

Gynecology   The branch of medicine which deals with women's diseases.

Homosexuality   Sexual attraction between members of the same sex.

Incest   Sexual intercourse between closely related persons such as father and daughter.

Infertility   Inability to conceive children.

Labor   Regular contractions of the uterus leading to childbirth.

Leiomyoma (fibroid)   A noncancerous tumor of the uterus composed of muscle cells.

Leprosy   A chronic disease which usually causes disfiguring of skin areas. It is a contagious disease caused by the microorganism, *Mycobacterium leprae.*

Lymphogranuloma venerum A venereal disease caused by a virus.

Mania An emotional state characterized by a severe overreaction of the emotions often leading to violent behavior.

Masturbation Autoerotic sexual stimulation.

Meningitis Inflammation of the coverings of the brain or spinal cord.

Menopause The general period in the life of a woman when ovulation and menstruation cease and when the lessening of hormonal activity produces the well-known signs of aging.

Menorrhagia Abnormally heavy menstrual flow.

Menstruation Periodic uterine bleeding in women of childbearing age.

Midwives Women competent in assisting in childbirth.

Miscarriage The expulsion of a fetus from the uterus before it has achieved adequate maturity for survival.

Monozygote In the case of twins, refers to both infants developing from the same egg.

Obstetrics The branch of medicine which deals with pregnancy, labor, and delivery.

Orthopedics That area of medicine concerned with bone and joint disease.

Ovulate To produce an egg from the ovary.

Paralysis The loss of ability to move a part of the body.

Paraplegia Paralysis of both legs.

Pituitary gland A small gland located near the base of the brain. It produces hormones which actuate other glands such as the thyroid and adrenal. It also secretes growth hormone—which if overly produced causes gigantism.

Placenta The organ (commonly called the "afterbirth") which grows attached to the inside of the uterus during pregnancy and through which nutrients and other materials are passed between the mother and fetus.

Polio A viral infection causing varying degrees of paralysis.

Polydactyly Condition of having an excessive number of fingers or toes.

Polygamy Having more than one spouse at the same time.

Psychophonasthenia Weakness or difficulty in speech caused by emotional problems.

Psychosis A general term for the more serious of mental illnesses. It usually refers to the situation in which a person loses contact with reality.

Quarantine The isolation of a person, animal, or object which harbors an infectious disease.

Retinitis Inflammation of the retina—the vision-receiving area of the eye—leading to various degrees of blindness.

Semen The male ejaculate which contains sperm.

Stroke Loss of function in various parts of the body usually caused by a vascular leak or occlusion in the brain.

Syphilis A venereal disease caused by the microorganism, *Treponema pallidum.*

Taenia solium A tapeworm reaching six feet in length which is transmitted to the human through the ingestion of poorly cooked pork meat.

Trachoma A viral infection of the external surfaces of the eye.

Trichinella spiralis A parasite which is transmitted to man most often through the ingestion of poorly cooked pork meat. It encysts in muscle.

Trichomonas vaginalis A protozoa which infects the vagina. Usually transmitted venereally.

Tuberculosis A chronic infectious disease often affecting the lungs, bones, or urinary-generative tracts. It is caused by the microorganism, *Bacillus tuberculosis.*

Venereal disease Any one of several infectious diseases transmitted through sexual relations.

Weaning The time when a child is no longer permitted to breast-feed.

Wet nurses Women employed to breast-feed infants other than their own.

A CHRONOLOGY
OF BIBLICAL MEDICINE

This is intended as a general guide for the reader who should recognize that some of these dates are arbitrary since scholars are not always in agreement for specific events.

Creation Accounts
 Adam, Eve

The Great Flood
 Noah, Divine Catastrophe

The Abraham Era
 Circumcision
 Jacob, Esau

Code of Hammurabi   *circa* 1950 B.C.
 Laws for Babylonian Cult Healers

Egyptian Medicine   The centuries before
 Mummification, Medical Papyri   and after the Exodus

The Exodus of Israel From Egypt   *circa* 1450 B.C.
 Moses
 Levitical (Mosaic) Health Laws
 Ten Commandments
 Desert Wanderings

The Entry of Israel into Canaan   1405 B.C.
 Judges Rule
 Samson
 Jael and Sisera

The United Hebrew Monarchy   1091 - 931 B.C.
 Saul, his psychosis
 David and Goliath
 Solomon and his wisdom, medical sayings

The Divided Kingdom	*circa* 931 B.C.
Medical problems of Kings	
Asa, Joram, Hezekiah, and Zedekiah	
Elijah	*circa* 860 B.C.
Elisha	*circa* 825 B.C.
Assyrian Captivity of Israel	722 B.C.
Zedekiah	597 - 586 B.C.
Last King of Judah	
Blinded by Babylonians	
Babylonian Captivity of Judah	586 B.C.
Nebuchadnezzar, King of Babylon	
Daniel	
Hippocrates	460 - 350 B.C.
Hippocratic Oath epitomized the centuries	
of medicine dominated by Greek thought	
Nehemiah	*circa* 440 B.C.
Governorship	
Birth of Christ	5 - 4 B.C.
Baptism of Christ	A.D. 27
Christ, the Master Healer, spends three	
and one half years in public teaching,	
healing, and raising the dead	
Crucifixion, Burial, and Resurrection	A.D. 31
Stoning of Stephen	A.D. 34
Rise of the Christian Church	
Paul's blindness and healing	
missionary travels	
Luke the Physician	
Work of the Apostles	
healings and faith concept	
Roman Destruction of Jerusalem by Titus	A.D. 70

INDEX